SpringerBriefs in Public Health

Child Health

Series Editor

Angelo P. Giardino

For further volumes:
http://www.springer.com/series/11600

Rohit Shenoi · Faria Pereira · Joyce Li
Angelo P. Giardino

The Complete Resource on Pediatric Office Emergency Preparedness

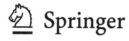 Springer

Rohit Shenoi
Faria Pereira
Texas Children's Hospital
Houston
TX
USA

Joyce Li
Boston Children's Hospital
Boston
MA
USA

Angelo P. Giardino
Texas Children's Health Plan
Houston
TX
USA

Additional material to this book can be downloaded from http://extras.springer.com/11600.

ISSN 2192-3698   ISSN 2192-3701   (electronic)
ISBN 978-1-4614-6903-2   ISBN 978-1-4614-6904-9   (eBook)
DOI 10.1007/978-1-4614-6904-9
Springer New York Heidelberg Dordrecht London

Library of Congress Control Number: 2013934721

© The Author(s) 2013
This work is subject to copyright. All rights are reserved by the Publisher, whether the whole or part of the material is concerned, specifically the rights of translation, reprinting, reuse of illustrations, recitation, broadcasting, reproduction on microfilms or in any other physical way, and transmission or information storage and retrieval, electronic adaptation, computer software, or by similar or dissimilar methodology now known or hereafter developed. Exempted from this legal reservation are brief excerpts in connection with reviews or scholarly analysis or material supplied specifically for the purpose of being entered and executed on a computer system, for exclusive use by the purchaser of the work. Duplication of this publication or parts thereof is permitted only under the provisions of the Copyright Law of the Publisher's location, in its current version, and permission for use must always be obtained from Springer. Permissions for use may be obtained through RightsLink at the Copyright Clearance Center. Violations are liable to prosecution under the respective Copyright Law.
The use of general descriptive names, registered names, trademarks, service marks, etc. in this publication does not imply, even in the absence of a specific statement, that such names are exempt from the relevant protective laws and regulations and therefore free for general use.
While the advice and information in this book are believed to be true and accurate at the date of publication, neither the authors nor the editors nor the publisher can accept any legal responsibility for any errors or omissions that may be made. The publisher makes no warranty, express or implied, with respect to the material contained herein.

Printed on acid-free paper

Springer is part of Springer Science+Business Media (www.springer.com)

We dedicate this work to Dr. Joan E. Shook, colleague, mentor, teacher, and tireless child advocate whose efforts over the past 25 years to improve emergency medical services for children has inspired us to work diligently to create educational programs that will assist office-based clinicians to be as prepared as possible for seriously ill and injured children who may present to requiring emergency care

Preface

Role of Primary Care Pediatrician in Dealing with Office Emergency Preparedness

The primary care pediatrician is an important link in the continuum of care of the critically ill and injured child from the point of presentation through stabilization, transport, definitive care, and finally rehabilitation. Patients may seek emergency care at the office because of the pre-existing trust and rapport with their primary care provider. Stabilizing the ill child in the office and early access to the Emergency Medical Services (EMS), are vital to ensure positive results. In 1993, the Institute of Medicine's Committee on Pediatric Emergency Medical Services issued a comprehensive set of recommendations intended to promote ideal Emergency Medical Services for Children (EMS-C) and part of this envisioned ideal system deals with the providers who see the seriously ill or injured child prior to definitive care available in a Pediatric Emergency Department. Understanding the resources available to the primary care pediatrician in the typical office setting and their limitations is also important in the education of their patients and their parents in the early recognition of emergency conditions and their prevention.

The American Academy of Pediatrics' Committee on Pediatric Emergency Medicine in 2007 issued a policy statement dealing with preparation for the potential for office-based emergency care and among the eight explicit recommendations three bear special attention and form the impetus for this book. The three paraphrased below are:

- #2 Develop an organized plan for the office to respond to an emergency;
- #5 Develop a plan for training and education for the office providers and staff;
- #6 Practice skills by doing mock codes in the office setting at least twice a year.

In the pages and videos that follow, we have provided you with practical tools and materials to step through an organized process to assess your office's current level of emergency preparedness, to develop a training and education plan for you and your office staff, list algorithms to follow around supplies, medications and skills necessary to respond to the seriously ill or injured child, while the EMS is active and until they arrive, and finally the scripts and videos that should help you conduct drills and mock codes so that you and your staff develop a level of confidence and expertise at doing your initial part of handling the emergency situation for a child in your office.

So, How Best to Utilize This Resource?

The Complete Resource on Pediatric Office Emergency Preparedness is meant to be a practical resource for the clinician and office manager in the pediatric primary care setting. Our intent is to provide you with the overview material, detailed practical clinical information, and an educational approach that will help you and your office team understand the content and gain experience in practice sessions so that on those rare occasions when an office emergency situation arises, you will be able to competently go through the steps of assessment, response, and transfer of the pediatric patient to the appropriate level of care. Towards that end, Chap. 1 provides an overview of the emergency medical response system and the role of the primary care office within that system. Chapter 2 contains the detailed clinical information, in the form of protocols and text around commonly encountered office-based emergencies as well as listing necessary equipment and medications that ought to be available to handle these emergencies. Chapter 3 provides the educational framework and training materials complete with mock code scripts, video material, and pre and post tests, to make the training sessions led by the clinician as valuable as possible. Chapter 4 provides a continuous quality improvement approach to how the modern office can approach its effort to prepare for potential office-based emergencies over time with an eye towards monitoring the office's efforts and improving in its level of preparedness. Finally, with the family's needs front and center in our minds, Chap. 5 provides basic information about how to include families in the preparation effort in the event their child needs emergency care. Ideally, the clinical and office manager who are organizing this effort would read the book through its entirety and then will use the content in Chap. 2 protocol and text to guide the training outlined in Chap. 3 and the quality improvement process described in Chap. 4. The videos provide a visual media adjunct that may make the training more engaging and feel more realistic.

Rohit Shenoi
Faria Pereira
Joyce Li
Angelo P. Giardino

References

American Academy of Pediatrics. (2007). Preparation for emergencies in the offices of pediatricians and pediatric primary care providers. Committee on pediatric emergency medicine. *Pediatrics, 120*, 200–212.

Durch, J. S., & Lohr, K. N. (Eds.). (1993). National Research Council. *Emergency Medical Services for Children*. Washington, DC: The National Academies Press.

Acknowledgments

The authors express gratitude to the Baylor College of Medicine, Academy of Distinguished Educators for initial grant funding to support the design of this handbook and the filming of the videos. Special thanks to Jim Shanahan, Jesus Chavez, Jr., Julie Eaves, C. Valerie Vance, Joanne Cummings, RN, and Lilianna Velasquez for assistance with the video production. We appreciate Dr. Richard Byrd at Kelsey-Seybold Clinics, Houston and Kay Tittle, President Texas Children's Pediatrics, for their assistance with setting up office preparedness educational experiences during which we could pilot and refine our work. Finally, we thank Kimberly A. Heffernan for her help in procuring the respiratory equipment and for demonstrating various respiratory-related techniques.

Contents

Abstract

Primary care practitioners recognize the need for emergency preparedness but face the challenges of a busy practice and infrequent opportunities to manage and coordinate the care of critically ill or injured children who may present to their office. During emergencies, providers and their staff are called on to work efficiently as a "code-team" which may be a source of considerable apprehension. Current resources to enhance pediatric emergency preparedness may not be suited for most office-based pediatricians.

This multi-component, multi-media educational resource consists of a handbook that describes key knowledge concepts, skills and up-to-date algorithms pertaining to important pediatric office emergencies; a series of learning videos of case vignettes that highlight both non-preferred and preferred management of common office emergencies; and a knowledge assessment module that can be used to test the learner's knowledge of pediatric office emergencies.

The authors supported by peer review and input from top specialists in Pediatric Emergency Medicine at the Baylor College of Medicine offer a comprehensive educational resource on pediatric office emergency preparedness devoted exclusively to the practicing primary care health care provider and his/her team. This unique reference guide contains a wealth of information and resources in a compact and practical form. It presents the most important knowledge, skills, office resources and team interactions required by practitioners to successfully treat pediatric emergencies in the office.

Chapter 1
Community Partnerships in Pediatric Office Emergency Preparedness

1.1 Role of Primary Care Provider in Emergency Medical Services for Children

Serving as the child's medical home, the primary care pediatrician (PCP) is responsible for health maintenance, well child care and for the coordination of care of sick and injured children with emergency medical services (EMS), hospital, and rehabilitation services.

At a community level, the primary care provider (PCP) performs different roles when providing emergency medical services for children (EMSC). These include educator, triage officer, provider of emergency care, consultant, advocate for children and participant in disaster management. As an educator, the PCP provides anticipatory guidance to families and educates them on illness and injury prevention. By being aware of the levels of emergency care and resources available in the community, the pediatrician can direct patients to the appropriate facilities for treatment. If emergencies occur in the office, the physician and office staff will stabilize and then transfer the child to the hospital. Almost 90 % of children requiring emergency care are treated in general hospitals. The PCP, as a consultant and child advocate, can provide important advice to his/her adult colleagues on the care of children. This includes transfer and treatments protocols, caring for children with special health care needs, the types of equipment and supplies required in pediatric emergency care and ongoing education in pediatric emergencies. Finally, the pediatrician will assist the community at large during the planning, preparation, and medical response during disasters (Seidel and Knapp 2000).

1.2 Primary Care Providers and EMS

The pediatric advanced life support (PALS) chain of survival is a sequence of interventions that was developed by the American Heart Association to reduce morbidity and mortality in children. It consists of: (1) prevention of injury and

R. Shenoi et al., *The Complete Resource on Pediatric Office Emergency Preparedness*, SpringerBriefs in Child Health, DOI: 10.1007/978-1-4614-6904-9_1, © The Author(s) 2013

death, (2) early recognition of cardiac arrest and effective cardiopulmonary resuscitation (CPR), (3) early activation of EMS, and (4) early advanced life support.

Since primary care providers will access EMS during emergencies, it is important for them to know the levels and capabilities of an EMS response. EMS services are administered and regulated at the state level. Though these services vary from state to state, there are several features that are common in most US states. This chapter will briefly review aspects of the EMS component in the chain of survival.

1.2.1 EMS Levels of Service

There are different levels of EMS response and they may vary by jurisdiction. However, the technical capabilities of the EMS personnel at the respective levels of EMS response are fairly uniform. For example, in a tiered response, there are first responders who render on-scene emergency care while awaiting additional EMS response. The next level of response involves a Basic EMT (BLS transport) who is skilled in basic life support (BLS), basic trauma care, and the use of an automated external defibrillator (AED). Paramedics (ALS transport) are the most skilled. They are trained in advanced life support skills through Advanced Cardiac Life Support (ACLS) and PALS and can perform life-saving procedures such as endotracheal intubation, intravenous or intra-osseous access. Not all states have a tiered response system, for example, in a rural setting, they may not have a tiered response due to staffing and availability of the provider type, but the definition of the personnel levels is usually similar across states.

When transporting a patient from a primary care clinic to the emergency department, you can call 911 for emergent situations or arrange for specific BLS or ALS transport. You should consider the skill level of the EMS providers in relation to the child's emergency condition and its potential for worsening when deciding which level of transport to request. Refer to the table below for the capabilities of each level of responders (Table 1.1).

Obtaining EMS access:

1. Call 911 or universal emergency number
2. Specify medical emergency
3. Inform accurate address
4. Specify specialized care needed (ALS)
5. Patient's age, condition, and vital signs
6. Indicate destination hospital.

Your local EMS:

As mentioned previously, the overall EMS structure and organization can vary between regions. For instance, in some jurisdictions, the EMS is in constant touch with a base hospital and/or supervising physician (**on-line control**). Elsewhere, EMS operates solely by written protocols (**off-line control**) with no active

Table 1.1 Skill levels of EMS responders

Provider	Scope of practice
First responder/emergency medical responder	• Initial history and physical exam
	• Remove patient from immediate danger
	• CPR and bag-mask ventilation
	• Operate an AED
	• Oxygen administration
	• Insert oropharyngeal airway
	• Suction airway
	• Apply direct pressure for control of bleeding and bandaging
	• Provide manual C-spine and fracture stabilization
	• Administer unit dose autoinjectors (e.g., EpiPen)
	• Assist uncomplicated delivery of newborn
Emergency medical technician-basic (EMT-B)/emergency medical technician	*As for first responder and*:
	• Perform basic on-scene triage
	• Access and extricate trapped victims
	• Apply traction splint
	• Perform spine immobilization (C-spine and backboard)
	• Apply tourniquet
	• Apply pneumatic antishock garment if indicated
	• Irrigate eyes
	• Basic burn management
	• Basic poisoning management (administration of activated charcoal)
	• Assist patient in taking their own prescribed medications (e.g., nitroglycerin SL)
	• Administration of limited oral medications (e.g., aspirin and glucose paste)
	• Assist complicated delivery of newborn
Emergency medical technician-intermediate (EMT-I)/advanced emergency medical technician	*As for first responder*, EMT-B and:
	• Orotracheal intubation or placement of multi-lumen airway
	• Suction already intubated patients
	• Peripheral IV access or IO access
	• Administer IV fluids
	• Administer limited medications (e.g., nitroglycerine SL, IM or SC epinephrine, IV dextrose, IM or IV naloxone)
	• Administer inhaled beta agonists

(continued)

Table 1.1 (continued)

Provider	Scope of practice
Emergency medical technician-paramedic (EMT-P)	*As for first responder*, EMT-B and EMT-I and: • Nasotracheal intubation of adults • Surgical airway • Chest decompression • Advanced rhythm interpretation • Manual ventricular defibrillation of adults and children • Vagal maneuvers • Synchronized cardioversion • Transcutaneous pacing • Comprehensive pharmacologic intervention • Central line infusions • Advanced triage • Straightening of select fractures and reducing dislocations if neurovascular compromise is evident • Advanced burn/ingestion management • Advanced newborn resuscitation

Sirbaugh and Meckler (2012)

physician input at the time of the emergency. You would have to call your local EMS to find out on which system they operate. We have provided a list of questions that will help you understand how your local EMS works and what to expect should you need their services during an in-office emergency. You can call your local fire department's non-urgent number to find out who oversees your local EMS.

Questions to ask about your EMS:

1. Under which EMS jurisdiction does your office lie?
2. Is it a volunteer, public, or private agency?
3. Does your area have an enhanced 911 capability? (can establish address of caller)
4. Is computer-aided dispatch used? (EMS operator used algorithm)
5. Is there a tiered response? (i.e., use of basic, intermediate, and paramedics)
6. Is there online or offline control? (physician supervision)
7. What pediatric training do the EMTs have? PALS?
8. Are Paramedics capable of inserting advanced airway? [endotracheal tube (ETT) and Laryngeal mask airway (LMA)]

1.2.2 Summary

Your office serves as the medical home for your patients. Families and patients will rely on you during times of medical crisis for direction and assistance. It is imperative that you develop and act on a plan to handle medical emergencies in your office. Gaining an appropriate understanding of your local EMS and community partners will assist in you providing the best possible care for your patients.

References

Sirbaugh, P. E., & Meckler, G. (2012). *Prehospital pediatrics and emergency medical services (EMS)*. Up to date, Inc. 2012.
Seidel, J. S., & Knapp, J. F. (2000). *Role of primary-care physician in EMS-C Childhood emergencies in the office, hospital and community Organizing systems of care* (pp. 3–8). Elk Grove Village, IL: American Academy of Pediatrics.

Chapter 2
The Office Emergency Response

Pediatric office emergencies are common and occur about once or twice per month. In urban areas, practices may encounter emergencies more often. About one patient per week may need to be transferred to a hospital's emergency department for evaluation and treatment. The varying numbers suggest the lack of an operational definition of what constitutes a pediatric office emergency. To be labeled an emergency condition, does it mean that a child needs to be transferred to the emergency department? Alternatively, does the child need to be acutely resuscitated in the clinic to call it an office emergency? In pondering over this question, the primary health provider should understand that the patient's disease process is a continuum. Acute deterioration may occur suddenly at an unexpected time and when optimal resources may not be available. This section will discuss the response to a pediatric office emergency.

Pediatric practices are ill prepared to handle office emergencies (Flores and Weinstock 1996; Walsh-Kelly et al. 2004; Shetty et al. 1998; Santillanes et al. 2006). Common problems that are faced by pediatricians include the following: inability of office staff to identify a sick child, poor triage policy, improper facility preparation, inadequate and improperly stored equipment and medications, inadequate knowledge and skills in pediatric emergency care, and poor team dynamics and role playing.

Some of the excuses given by pediatricians when asked why they are not well prepared in handling medical emergencies in the office are as follows:

1. "Emergencies are not common!" Emergencies may vary in frequency and show a seasonal variation. However, one poorly managed office emergency is one too many for a provider whose aim is to provide the best care for his or her patients.
2. "I practice in an urban area and the EMS personnel will respond quickly!" EMS is an excellent resource for stabilizing and transporting very ill or injured children to the hospital. However, in urban areas, they may take at least 7–10 min to arrive at the office. In remote areas, the delay may be longer. Effective life-saving treatment should never be delayed.
3. "Having life-saving equipment may increase my liability!" The inability to provide effective resuscitation occurs when providers lack experience and skills. Liability will increase when substandard care is provided.

R. Shenoi et al., *The Complete Resource on Pediatric Office Emergency Preparedness*, SpringerBriefs in Child Health, DOI: 10.1007/978-1-4614-6904-9_2, © The Author(s) 2013

4. "Resuscitation equipment may be expensive!" Some types of life-saving equipment are expensive, such as the color-coded resuscitation carts with disposable equipment. However, most of the basic life support equipment is not expensive.

Types of Office Emergencies

The common pediatric office emergencies include respiratory distress due to asthma, bronchiolitis or pneumonia, seizures, shock due to hypovolemia (usually dehydration) or sepsis or anaphylaxis, diabetic ketoacidosis, head injury with altered mental status, psychosocial emergencies (child abuse and domestic violence, depression with suicidal intent). Rare causes include acute traumatic conditions with hemorrhage, choking, respiratory failure with apnea, and cardiac arrest.

Organization of a Pediatric Office Emergency Response

These are the steps that need to be taken to ensure a quick and effective response to pediatric office emergencies:

1. Early recognition of a sick child in the clinic.
2. Activation of EMS.
3. Transfer child to the treatment room.
4. Delineation of staff roles in emergency treatment area.
5. Emergency response.
6. Transfer care to EMS personnel with code sheet.

2.1 Triage: Recognition of Emergency by Reception Area or Secretarial Staff and Nursing Staff

The optimal management of a critically ill child begins with efficient and accurate triage performed by the clinic nurse either when a caregiver calls in by telephone or when the child presents to the clinic (see fig. 2.1). Office staff should be well versed in performing triage. In coming to the best decision, the provider must obtain key historical information about the child's condition and consider whether a treatment delay is likely to be harmful to the child. They should err on the side of caution. There are excellent resources available on pediatric triage (Schmitt 2010). Based on their triage, they should correctly instruct caregivers who call in, whether to bring the ill child to the office, to proceed directly to the emergency department, or to summon emergency medical services (EMS).

A caregiver who is calling into the office should hang up and **call EMS if**

1. The child has a potentially life-threatening medical condition.
2. The child is too unstable to transport by private conveyance.
3. There is a risk of further injury if the child is moved (e.g., trauma).
4. The clinic personnel do not have the requisite life support skills or equipment to effectively manage the patient.

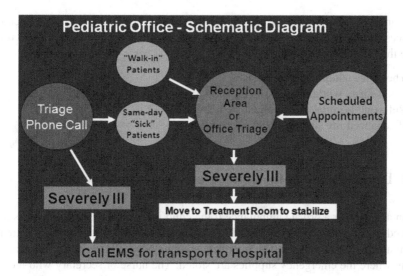

Fig. 2.1   The diagram illustrates the different pathways in which a severely ill child may be recognized in the office setting

At the office, the front-desk personnel are often the first people to assess a child. They, as well as the nursing staff, should be taught how to rapidly recognize a critically ill child. This rapid assessment can be easily taught by the physician and should include the following:

Skin   How does the child look? (pale, bluish or dusky, mottled or petechiae/rash)

Breathing   What is the rate? (rapid or slow)What is the effort? (chest retractions, nasal flaring, head bobbing)

Appearance   How is the child responding to the environment? (somnolent, poorly aroused, agitated)

A child who demonstrates any of these findings is likely to be very ill. The child should be rapidly moved to the treatment area for further assessment and stabilization and then transferred to the emergency department by EMS. Other conditions which warrant immediate assessment are active seizures, vomiting after a head injury, or uncontrolled bleeding. If the office is busy, the nurse and office staff should periodically monitor the waiting room patients to check whether their condition has worsened.

2.2 Activation of EMS

Office staff must be aware how to access emergency services if a critically ill child presents to the clinic when a physician is not present. At least one of the providers in the office should be able to provide basic life support until EMS arrives.

A written office protocol on who needs to access EMS and under what circum-stances should be prepared ahead of time. The person accessing EMS should pro-vide the following information:

1. The office address and location.
2. Child's age, working assessment, and vital signs.
3. Referring hospital if the patient's condition allows it.
4. If advanced life support skills are needed.

2.3 Transfer Patient to Appropriate Treatment Area

Even as EMS (or a private ambulance if the child is less severely ill) is being sum-moned to the clinic, the critically ill child should be moved quickly to the treat-ment area in a safe manner. The treatment area may be a treatment or examination room where the emergency supplies are stored. The nurse or secretary who recog-nized the emergency should immediately notify the physician and other members of the clinic response team.

2.4 Delineation of Staff Roles in Treatment Area

The office management should develop a written office protocol to specify the roles of each member of the office response team. The usual roles for response team members are as follows:

Physician	The physician directs the "code," manages the airway, and performs life support procedures such as bag and mask ventilation and intra-osseous access. He/she will organize the team, monitor performance and serve as a backup for inadequacies in response team members, verbalize the "mental model" (a concise description of the patient's medical problems), and ensure that the emergency response is being run smoothly
Nurse	The nurse will obtain intravenous access and prepare and administer medications and fluids
Medical Assistant	The assistant will assist the physician in procedures, perform chest compressions if needed, and assist the nurse in obtaining supplies
Secretary	The secretary is responsible for activating the EMS, communicating with the family, recording events, and copying the medical chart for the referring hospital

An effective response team will demonstrate excellent resuscitation skills and medical expertise, good communication, and superior team dynamics. Each member will be aware of their roles and responsibilities. They will acknowledge and read back orders made by the team leader (physician) and voice their concerns if there are any discrepancies. All members of the response team will work with a single purpose of effectively stabilizing the critically ill child and transferring care to EMS.

2.5 Emergency Response

Once the child is in the treatment room, the provider should perform an immediate assessment of the airway, breathing, and circulatory status of the patient. The questions to ask are as follows:

1. Is the child in respiratory distress? If so, is it moderately severe or very severe? Severe air hunger is manifest by deep chest retractions, audible inspiratory stridor, absent air entry in the lungs, cyanosis, grunting, and somnolence.
2. Is the airway clear and patent with good air entry bilaterally? If so, the child should be carefully observed for future deterioration. Is the air flow to the lungs obstructed due to patient position or upper airway obstruction (caused by flexion of the neck, large tongue, or secretions)? If so, a head tilt and jaw thrust or suctioning of the oropharynx may alleviate the patient's problems. Does the child have shallow or irregular breaths or is altogether apneic? If so, the child requires bag and mask ventilation and EMS need to be summoned. It is safe to manually ventilate a child using an Ambu-bag and mask with high-flow oxygen for a brief period until EMS arrive.
3. Is the child in circulatory shock? If so, is it compensated (normal blood pressure) or uncompensated (low systolic blood pressure for age)? Weak central pulses with absent peripheral pulses with signs of inadequate tissue perfusion such as lethargy, altered mental status, oliguria, pallor, mottled skin, and delayed capillary refill suggest hypotensive or uncompensated shock. These patients are critically ill and deteriorate very rapidly.
4. What is the mental status of the child? A quick assessment of consciousness should be performed using the AVPU method (A = Alert; V = responds to Voice; P = responds to Pain; and U = Unconscious). Alternatively, the Glasgow Coma Scale can be used to more accurately determine the level of consciousness.
5. What is the weight of the patient in kilograms? If this has not been done earlier, you may use a color-coded length-based resuscitation tape (*Broselow tape*) to get an approximate weight of the child. With the child in a recumbent position, hold one end of the tape against the top of the head and mark the tape at the level of the feet. Use this mark to obtain the weight, equipment sizes, and doses of the resuscitation medications that may be required.

Resuscitation must be based on repeated clinical assessments and observing the response to various resuscitative interventions. The reader is referred to emergency treatment protocols for managing specific conditions which are located elsewhere in the book.

2.6 Transfer Care to EMS Unit with Code Sheet

The physician should hand over care of the patient to EMS personnel when they arrive. A concise history of the patient's medical symptoms and signs, interventions performed, and the response to these interventions should be mentioned. Specifically, the physician should mention the following:

1. Age and sex of the child.
2. Presenting symptoms.
3. Relevant past history including allergies.
4. Vital signs at presentation with estimated or correct weight in kilograms.
5. Type of measures performed and the response to them.
6. All drugs and fluids that were given, their dose, and mode of administration (code log), see Fig. 2.2.
7. The transferring hospital if the condition of the child allows it.
8. Call and speak to the physician at receiving hospital's emergency department alerting him/her of the patient transfer.

2.7 Sample Office Emergency Policy

In the event of a respiratory and/or cardiac or impending arrest, the "911" emergency system should be initiated.

1.00   General Information

    1.10   Office staff should ensure that the physician on-site is notified of the event

    1.20   All persons who experience cardiac or respiratory arrest or pending failure should have resuscitation attempted by using the American Heart Association protocol for basic life support

    1.30   All providers and clinical office staff should have at a minimum, a current AHA basic life support (BLS) for healthcare provider course card

    1.40   Patient requiring higher-level care must be transported by EMS only, except those practices located on a hospital campus with written protocols for provider-assisted transfer

    1.50   Each office should have the following emergency supplies, medications, or physician-determined alternatives:

    Emergency Supplies:
    Airway kit containing oropharyngeal airway sizes for infant through adult
    OR
    Airways oral, infant through adult sizes, disposable—minimum of 2 each
    Ambu-bags and mask—infant, disposable—minimum of 2

MONTH	DAY	YEAR	CODE START TIME	CPR TIME	CODE END TIME	ALLERGIES		
911 CALLED	EMS ARRIVE	EMS DEPART	EMS COMPANY	EMT		EMT		CODE CALLED

TEAM	NAME		TIME	TEAM	NAME		TIME	TEAM	NAME		TIME
PHYSICIAN				RN/LVN							
PHYSICIAN				MA							
RN/LVN				MA							

VITAL SIGNS								RESPIRATORY PROCEDURES					
Time								METHOD	TIME	METHOD	TIME	SIZE	
B/P								Oxygen ____ L/min		Ambu Bag			
Pulse								Nasal Cannula		Oral Airway			
Respiration								Mask		Suction			
Temperature								LAB WORK					
Pulse Ox													

INTRAVENOUS THERAPY					Solution / Amount						
Type	Size	Site	Started	By Who	Solution	Started	Rate	By Who		Amount In	
IV											
IO											

MEDICATIONS	Time	Amount Route	By Who	Time	Amount Route	By Who	MEDICATIONS	Time	Amount	Route	By Who
Epinephrine 1:10000							Ceftriaxone				
Epinephrine 1:1000							Dexamethasone				
Epi Pen Jr							Dextrose 25%				
Epi Pen							Dextrose 50%				
Diazepam							Diphenhydramine				

TIME	OTHER EVENTS		PATIENT VARIABLES	
			Survived	
			Expired	
			Transfer to:	
	Recorder Signature			Date:
	Physician Signature			Date:

Name:
DOB:
MR#:

Fig. 2.2 Code log. Adapted and permission courtesy of Texas Children's Pediatrics, Houston, Texas

Ambu-bags and mask—child, disposable—minimum of 2
Ambu-bags and mask—adult, disposable—minimum of 2
Automated external defibrillator (AED)
Automated external defibrillator (AED) electrode pads (adults and
      pediatric)—2 each
Backboard/cardiac arrest board
Fluid resuscitation access supplies:
      Intraosseous (IO) needles (18, 15)—minimum of 2 each
      *** AND/OR ***

Intravenous (IV) catheters in age-appropriate sizes (24, 22, 20)—minimum of 2 each

Intravenous (IV) start kit—minimum of 2

Intravenous (IV) tubing with buretrol—minimum of 2

Venous access support supplies:

Armboards (2 × 4, 2 × 9)—minimum of 2 each

Sterile dressing materials (transparent tape, 2 × 2 gauze, 4 × 4 gauze, 2″ gauze wrap)

Oxygen administration supplies:

Oxygen masks for pediatric, adult (simple)—minimum of 2 each

Oxygen masks for pediatric, adult (non-rebreather)—minimum of 2 each

Portable oxygen

Pediatric measuring tape for emergency medication dosage (Broselow™ tape 2011 or current version)

Suctioning equipment:

Portable suction machine

Bulb syringe—minimum of 2

Tonsil tip (Yankauer) suction catheter with tubing—minimum of 2

Suction catheters age-appropriate sizes (6, 8, 10, 12)—minimum of 2 each

Emergency Medications:

Ceftriaxone 1-gram vial—minimum of 2

Dexamethasone (4 mg/ml) 5-ml vial—minimum of 2

Dextrose 25 % (250 mg/mL) 10-mL syringe—minimum of 2

Dextrose 50 % (500 mg/mL) vial—minimum of 2

Diazepam: Graduated diazepam rectal dispensing mechanisms are permissible as long as the full range of dosing can be achieved

Diazepam 2.5 mg rectal suppository—minimum of 2

Diazepam 10 mg rectal suppository—minimum of 2

*** AND/OR ***

Diazepam (5 mg/mL) injectable vial—minimum of 2

Diphenhydramine (50 mg/mL) 1-mL vial—minimum of 2

Epinephrine:

Epinephrine 1:10000 (0.1 mg/1 mL) syringe—minimum of 2

Epinephrine 1:1000 (1 mg/1 mL) ampule—minimum of 2

EpiPen Jr 1:2000 (0.15 mg/0.3 mL)—minimum of 2 (at the practice's discretion)

EpiPen 1:1000 (0.3 mg/0.3 mL)—minimum of 2 (at the practice's discretion)

Normal saline 500 mL bag—minimum of 2

1.60   All emergency supplies and medications should be recorded using the PeopleSoft's supply ordering interface to replace used items

2.00   Response Personnel

    2.10   All physicians, licensed independent practitioners (PA, PNP), and clinical personnel (RN, LVN, MA) should report to the patient, so basic life support measures may be initiated
    2.20   The physician or licensed independent practitioner will direct personnel to initiate the "911."
    2.30   If physician or licensed independent practitioner is not present, any staff may initiate "911" service. The physician or licensed independent practitioner should be immediately notified. If during posted business hours, the patient should be allowed into the practice to await EMS transportation even if no medical staff are available
    2.40   Physician or licensed independent practitioner will direct staff to notify hospital of pending admission and assure next of kin is notified

3.00   Termination of CPR

    3.10   CPR should continue until "911" response team has arrived and assumed care

4.00   Documentation (EMR)

    4.10   Code log should be completed for each impending office emergency
            a. Original should be scanned into patient medical record
            b. Document ambulance transfer in patient medical record
            c. After scanning, shred original document
            d. Send copy to quality department for tracking and trending purposes

5.00   Automated External Defibrillators (AED)

    5.10   Usage
            a. An AED is a recognized tool used in conjunction with resuscitation and may be made available for use on all persons
            b. Follow current AHA standards and prompts of the AED
    5.20   Maintenance
            a. A service representative of the AED supplier shall be contacted immediately upon indication of the AED needing service as outlined by the AED operations' manual

6.00   Quality Assurance

    6.10   Emergency supplies will be checked on a monthly basis for accessibility and functionality. This assessment will be recorded on the practice's quality assurance log
    6.20   Quality department will develop a plan to measure competency and provide guidance to both provider and clinical staff members in the use of the emergency supplies and medications required within this policy
    6.30   Practice sites with after-hours care should check the emergency supplies daily

6.40   Emergency supplies will be accessible during office hours and appropriately secured after office hours

6.50   All ambulance transfers must be documented. A copy of the letter should be printed and sent with the ambulance service for transition of care to the receiving facility

7.00   Quality Review

7.10   Regular review of codes and ambulance transfers will be conducted as part of the quality improvement process by one or more practice advisory committees

Adapted and permission courtesy of Texas Children's Pediatrics, Houston, Texas.

2.8 Pediatric Office Emergency Protocols

Some pediatric office emergencies such as seizures or respiratory distress due to asthma, bronchiolitis, or croup are common. Other emergencies are sporadic and infrequent but nevertheless life-threatening. These include respiratory failure, sepsis, circulatory shock, choking, and anaphylaxis. Primary-care pediatricians should be well versed with up-to-date treatment protocols for all possible pediatric office emergencies.

2.8.1 Protocols for Common Pediatric Office Emergencies

2.8.1.1 Asthma

Asthma presents with recurrent episodes of wheezing, dyspnea, prolonged expiratory phase, and diminished air exchange secondary to narrowing of mid-sized to small airways. This leads to increased work of breathing with chest retractions, hypoxia (low oxygen saturations <93 %) and poor feeding. Status asthmaticus exists when there is a failure to respond to initial bronchodilator therapy (National Heart association 2007; Murphy et al. 2006; Clinical Guidelines 2012; Castro-Rodriguez and Rodrigo 2004; Rowe et al. 2007).

Severe asthma: Marked chest tightness, marked wheezing and retractions, cyanosis, inability to speak in sentences, hunched posture, and altered mental status.

Assessment	**ABC's**-Vital signs and pulse oximetry—circulatory and respiratory status
	Characterize degree of respiratory distress (Clinical Respiratory Score*)
	Respond appropriately per BLS/PALS protocols
	Onset of symptoms, current medications, risk factors for severe disease (below)
Management	
Oxygen	Administer **oxygen** to maintain SpO$_2$ to ≥92 %
	Nasal cannula, blow-by oxygen, face mask @ 5 L/min or
	Non-rebreather oxygen mask @ >10 L/min
Nebulized Broncho Dilators	**Albuterol 0.15 mg/kg (min. 2.5 mg; max: 5 mg)** in combination with
	Ipratropium (0.25 mg: <12 years; 0.5 mg: >12 years) in 2.5 cc saline
	May repeat every 20 min for 3 doses
	or
	Short-acting β-agonist (**albuterol MDI**) with valved spacer
	If mild: <2 years: 4 puffs; ≥2 years: 6 puffs 1 dose and reassess
	If worse: <2 years: 6 puffs; >2 years: 6–8 puffs Q20 min up to 3 doses
	If poor air entry and patient unable to cooperate, may administer
	1:1000 epinephrine 0.01 ml/kg SC (max: 0.3 cc)
Steroids	Administer **PO prednisolone 2 mg/kg** ASAP (max: 60 mg) or
	PO or IM dexamethasone 0.2 mg/kg (max: 10 mg)

Caution in cases with potential life-threatening asthma:

1. Previous intubation or ICU admission.
2. ≥ 2 hospitalizations or ≥ 3 ED visits in past year.
3. Use of >1 canister of short-acting beta-agonist per month.
4. Poor compliance and access to care.
5. Lack of perception of disease severity (parent or child).
6. Rapid disease progression.
7. Major psychosocial problems.

Transfer to ED/call EMS when

1. No improvement in initial three bronchodilator treatments.
2. Persisting low oxygen saturations (<94 %).
3. Marked increase work of breathing and exhaustion.
4. Poor mental status—somnolence, agitation, lethargy (Table 2.1).

Table 2.1 Clinical respiratory score

Clinical respiratory score (CRS)			
Assess	Score 0	Score 1	Score 2
Respiratory rate	<2 mos <50 2–12 mos <40 1–5 years <30 >5 years <20	<2 mos 50–60 2–12 mos 40–50 >1–5 years 30–40 >5 years 20–30	<2 mos >60 2–12 mos >50 >1–5 years >40 >5 years >30
Auscultation	Good air movement, scattered expiratory wheezing, loose rales/crackles	Depressed air movement, inspiratory and expiratory wheezes, or rales/crackles	Diminished or absent breath sounds, severe wheezing or rales/crackles or marked prolonged expiration
Use of accessory muscles	Mild to no use of accessory muscles. Mild to no retractions, nasal flaring on inspiration	Moderate intercostal retractions, mild to moderate use of accessory muscles, nasal flaring	Severe intercostal and substernal retractions, nasal flaring
Mental status	Normal to mildly irritable	Irritable, agitated, restless	Lethargic
Room air SpO_2	>95 %	90–95 %	<90 %
Color	Normal	Pale to normal	Cyanotic, dusky

(Add score from all rows to calculate total CRS score)

Clinical Respiratory Score * (CRS) in asthma exacerbations:

Mild exacerbation:	CRS: ≤ 3
Moderate exacerbation:	CRS: 4–6
Severe exacerbation:	CRS: 6–8

2.8.1.2 Blunt Head Trauma

Assessment:

1. Mechanism: Fall from significant height, motor vehicle crash, penetrating injury, or suspected inflicted injury.
2. Symptoms: Seizure, altered mental status or loss of consciousness, severe headache, persistent vomiting.
3. Vital Signs: Heart rate, respiratory rate, blood pressure, oxygen saturation, capillary refill.
4. Neurological Examination: Glasgow Coma Scale (GCS) (see Table 2.2) or AVPU* and neurological deficits.
5. Coexisting neck injury.

Indications for non-contrast CT head: (to rule out skull fracture and intracranial bleed)

1. Altered mental status (agitation, somnolence, repetitive questioning).
2. Loss of consciousness (more than a few seconds and associated with high-risk mechanism).
3. Seizure.
4. Persistent vomiting.
5. GCS 14 or less.
6. Focal neurological findings.
7. Signs of acute skull fracture or basilar skull fracture ("Raccoon eyes—periorbital ecchymosis," "Battle sign"—bruising in the mastoid area, blood tinged or clear drainage from nostrils or ears, hemotympanum).
8. Infant with boggy scalp swelling in the parietal, temporal, or occipital areas or with bulging fontanel.
9. Severe injury mechanisms: May be first observed for 4–6 h in the absence of any of the preceding findings.
   > Falls from >3 feet (under 2 years of age) or from >5 feet (above 2 years of age)
   > Head struck by high-impact object
   > Automobile–pedestrian crash
   > Fall from bicycle without helmet
   > Automobile crash with patient ejection, rollover, or death of another passenger
10. Suspicion of child abuse.

Management:

1. *NPO*.
2. *Cervical spine precautions*: Cervical collar and posterior spine board (backboard).
3. *Protect airway*: Recovery position if vomiting.
4. *Head-elevated position*: 30 °.

5. *Call EMS* if transport is necessary and to stabilize cervical spine.
6. *IV normal saline bolus* of 20 cc/kg if inadequate systemic perfusion.

Transfer to hospital/call EMS when patient has

1. Cardiorespiratory compromise.
2. Altered mental status.
3. Neurological deficits.
4. Neck injuries, multiple injuries, and non-accidental trauma.

Previously neurologically healthy children with minor closed head injury could be observed in the clinic, emergency department, hospital, or home under the care of a competent caregiver.

These patients should have

1. Normal mental status,
2. No abnormal or focal findings on neurological (including fundoscopic) examination,
3. No evidence of skull fracture (hemotympanum, basilar skull fracture, or palpable depression).

Neurologically normal patients with a normal cranial CT scan are at very low risk of subsequent deterioration.

Table 2.2 Glasgow coma score

Component	Response (Adult)	Response (Pediatric)	Score
Eye opening	Spontaneous	Spontaneous	4
	To command	To sound	3
	To pain	To pain	2
	None	None	1
Verbal response	Oriented	Age-appropriate vocalization, smile, or orientation to sound, interacts (coos, babbles), follows objects	5
	Confused, disoriented	Cries, irritable	4
	Inappropriate words	Cries to pain	3
	Incomprehensible sounds	Moans to pain	2
	None	None	1
Motor response	Obeys commands	Spontaneous movements (obeys verbal command)	6
	Localizes pain	Withdraws to touch (localizes pain)	5
	Withdraws	Withdraws to pain	4
	Abnormal flexion to pain (decorticate posture)	Abnormal flexion to pain (decorticate posture)	3
	Abnormal extension to pain (decerebrate posture)	Abnormal extension to pain (decerebrate posture)	2
	None	None	1

Kuppermann et al. (2009)

Glasgow Coma Score (GCS): Assign a score for the best response for each component and then add all three components for a composite GCS score (Table 2.2).

*AVPU—assessment of mental status (response to)
Alert
Voice
Pain
Unresponsive

2.8.1.3 Bronchiolitis

It is most commonly caused in infants by viral lower respiratory tract infection and is characterized by acute inflammation, edema, and necrosis of epithelial cells lining small airways, increased mucus production, and bronchospasm. The diagnosis is mainly clinical. The hallmark is increased respiratory rate and wheezing. Treatment is controversial, as efficacy has not been demonstrated consistently (Diagnosis and Management of Bronchiolitis 2006; Bronchiolitis Guideline Team, Cincinnati Children's Hospital Medical Center 2012; Viswanathan et al. 2003; Mansback et al. 2008; Levine et al. 2004).

Risk factors for severe disease:

1. Age <12 weeks
2. History of prematurity (<37 weeks)
3. Underlying cardiopulmonary disease
4. Others: Immunodeficiency, neurologic disease, congenital defects of airway

Severe disease:

Increased respiratory effort, grunting, nasal flaring, chest retractions.
Normal Respiratory Rates:
<2 months: < 50/min
2–12 months: <40/min
1–5 years: <30/min

Assessment:

1. Impact of respiratory symptoms on feeding and hydration.
2. Response if any to treatment.

Management:

ABCs	Assess cardiorespiratory status; evaluate Clinical Respiratory Score
	Reassess frequently
β-adrenergics	Single administration. Assess before and 1 h after treatment
(Albuterol/Levalbuterol)	**Albuterol (2.5 mg in 2.5 ml saline or 0.083 % vials)** nebulized solution or as MDI 90 mcg/inhalation: 4–6 puffs with spacer and mask
or	**or**
	Levalbuterol (0.63–1.25 mg/3 ml) nebulized solution or as MDI 45 mcg/inhalation: 2–4 puffs with spacer and mask

(If clinical response to albuterol or levalbuterol may administer every 4–6 h PRN)

α-adrenergics   Inhaled **racemic epinephrine (2.25 %)**
0.05 cc/kg/dose in 3 ml saline (max. 0.5 cc)

Nasal saline drops (0.65 %) 1–2 gtts TID PRN; **nasal suction** before feeds and breathing treatments and PRN

Contact isolation, hand decontamination, and no tobacco smoke exposure

Supplemental oxygen only if SpO_2 falls persistently <90 % in previously healthy infants. Discontinue O_2 if SpO_2 is ≥90 % and infant feeding well.

Hydration and fluids: IV fluids when respiratory rate >60–70/min with increased work of breathing. Continue breast-feeding if respiratory status permits.

Not useful: Ipratropium, corticosteroids, oral bronchodilators, chest physiotherapy

Antibiotics: If less than 60 days with fever—evaluate for serious bacterial infection/urinary tract infection. Use antibiotics only with specific indications of coexisting bacterial infection.

Transfer to ED/call EMS when

1. Persisting low oxygen saturations <90 %
2. Marked increase work of breathing and tachypnea (RR >60/min)
3. Poor feeding, lethargy, and dehydration
4. Apneic episodes

2.8.1.4 Cardiac Arrest

Cardiac arrest in children is usually a terminal event following respiratory failure and shock. Five to 15 % of cardiac arrests in children are caused by ventricular fibrillation and pulseless ventricular tachycardia (Fig. 2.3) (Kleinman et al. 2010a, b).

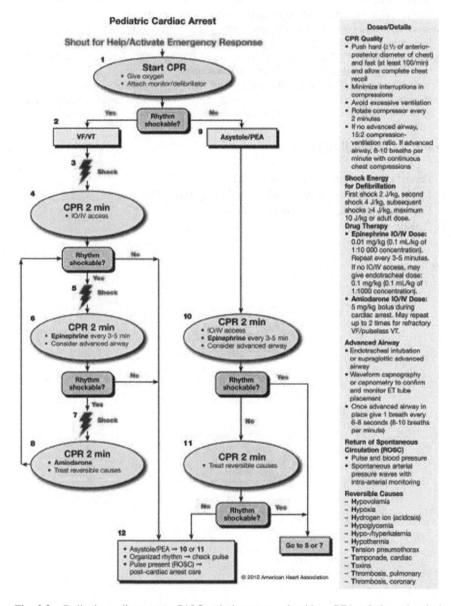

Fig. 2.3 Pediatric cardiac arrest—PALS pulseless arrest algorithm. *PEA* pulseless electrical activity. Permission pending. Reprinted with permission 2012 American Heart Guidelines for CPR and ECC. Part 14: Pediatric Advanced Life Support. *Circulation* 2010; 122 [supl 3]:S876–S908. ©2010 American Heart Association, Inc

2.8.1.5 Choking—Child

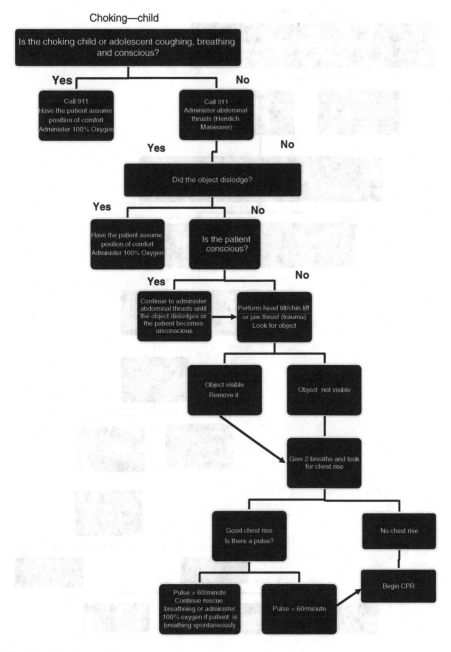

Fig. 2.4 Choking—child

2.8.1.6 Choking—Infant

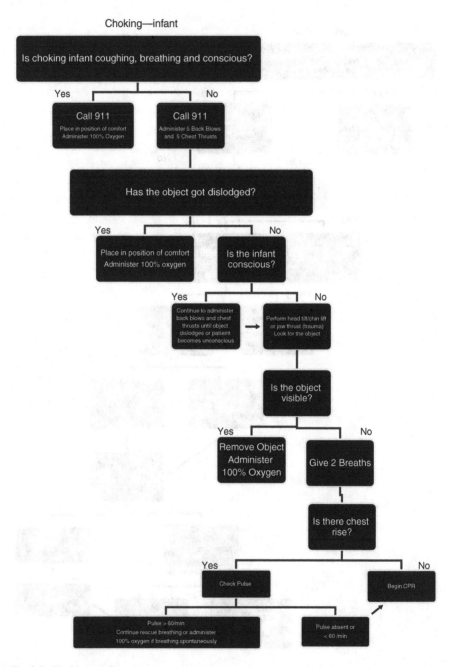

Fig. 2.5   Choking—infant

2.8.1.7 *Croup (Laryngotracheitis)*

It is a respiratory illness characterized by inspiratory stridor, barking cough, and hoarse voice. Fever may or may not be present. Infectious croup is usually viral in etiology, whereas spasmodic croup is not. Hypoxia results from severe airway obstruction (Table 2.3).

Assessment   ABCs, assess croup severity by *Westley Score*

Table 2.3 Westley score

Clinical sign	Points (range 0-17 points) 0 points	
Level of consciousness	Normal, including sleep	Disoriented = 5points
Cyanosis	None	Cyanosis with agitation = 4 points; cyanosis at rest = 5 points
Stridor	None	Stridor with agitation = 1 point; stridor at rest = 2 points
Air entry	Normal	Decreased = 1 point; markedly decreased = 2 points
Retractions	None	Mild = 1 point; moderate = 2 points; severe = 3 points

Mild croup: ≤2 points; *moderate croup: 3–7 points*; *severe croup: ≥8 points*

Management

Oxygen	Administer supplemental **oxygen** to maintain saturation >94 %
Stridor at rest	**Nebulized racemic epinephrine (2.25 %) 0.05 ml/kg** per dose (Max. dose 0.5 ml) in 3 ml saline
	OR
	Nebulized 0.5 ml/kg 1:1,000 L-epinephrine (max. dose: 5 ml) diluted in saline
	Observe for at least 2 h for rebound of croup symptoms
Steroids	Administer **dexamethasone PO or IM 0.6 mg/kg** (max. dose: 10 mg)
	May administer injectable preparation orally
Position	Assume position of comfort—in parent's arms
Respiratory Failure	(Signs: fatigue, listlessness, marked chest retractions, absent breath sounds, somnolence)
	Bag and Mask Ventilation
	Choose an endotracheal tube 0.5 to 1 mm smaller than indicated for intubation
Not helpful	Antibiotics
	β₂-agonists (albuterol)
	Antitussives and decongestants
	Humidified air

Transfer to ED/call EMS when

1. Fatigue and listlessness, marked retractions, decreased or absent breath sounds, somnolence
2. Stridor at rest unresponsive to racemic epinephrine
3. No response to treatment and patient has high fever with toxicity
4. Oxygen saturation <92 %
5. Cyanosis
6. Possible foreign body or caustic ingestion
7. Excessive drooling

2.8.1.8 Diabetic Ketoacidosis

Diabetic ketoacidosis (DKA) is a decrease in effective circulating insulin associated with increase in counter regulatory hormones (e.g., glucagon, catecholamines, cortisol, and growth hormone). Hyperglycemia and acidosis result in osmotic diuresis, dehydration, and electrolyte loss. The biochemical criteria include a blood glucose > 200 mg/dl; venous pH < 7.25 (arterial pH < 7.3); and/or bicarbonate <15 mmol/L. In the office, elevated blood glucose with glucosuria and ketonuria in the appropriate clinical setting is enough to suspect DKA and refer the child to the emergency department.

History:

1. New or established type 1 diabetes (IDDM)
2. Age
3. Concurrent illness
4. Estimated weight loss
5. Abdominal pain or vomiting
6. Altered mental status
7. Last dose Insulin: amount and time

Assessment:

1. Pulse rate, respiratory rate, blood pressure, temperature, weight, length.

Table 2.4 Formula to calculate body surface area

	Body surface area in M^2
5–10 kg	kg × 0.04 + 0.1
10–20 kg	kg × 0.03 + 0.2
20–40 kg	kg × 0.02 + 0.4
>40 kg	kg × 0.01 + 0.8

Calculate body surface area (Table 2.4)
2. Level of consciousness: AVPU or Glasgow Coma Scale, Kussmaul's breathing (rapid and/or deep sighing)
3. Dehydration: Cool skin, diaphoresis, weak pulses, delayed capillary refill, hypotension, oliguria, somnolence
4. Cerebral edema: Abnormal disk margins, inappropriately low heart rate, increase in BP, altered mental status

High-risk children:

1. Age <5 years
2. New onset IDDM

3. Altered mental status
4. Severe dehydration/shock, cardiac arrhythmias, or EKG changes
5. Glucose >800 mg/dl
6. Cerebral edema (inappropriately low heart rate, increase in BP, altered mental status)

Management: Goal is to stabilize and rapidly transfer to hospital for definitive (insulin and fluid) therapy

1. Immediate bedside blood glucose level.
2. Assess airway, place on monitor and pulse—oximeter.
3. Obtain IV access. If in shock, administer oxygen and fluid bolus (below).
4. *Lactated ringer* (*LR*) 10 ml/kg bolus over 1 h and if clinically indicated, repeat once (may use normal saline if LR is unavailable)
5. *Do not give* sodium bicarbonate
6. Total fluids: 2,500 ml/m^2/day (do not exceed 4,000 ml/m^2/day including bolus)

Transfer to hospital/call EMS when

1. Diagnosis of DKA suspected
2. Altered mental status
3. Dehydration and shock
4. Respiratory distress.

2.8.1.9 Seizures

Seizures are caused by abnormal and sustained electrical discharges from the cerebral neurons. Seizures may present as gaze abnormalities, lip-smacking, facial or limb twitching, and unresponsiveness in infants. Older children may demonstrate unilateral or generalized repetitive muscular contractions or stiffening of the limbs with unresponsiveness followed by hypotonia. Seizures may be associated with fever, hypoxia, metabolic causes including hypoglycemia, intracranial infection or bleeding, toxic ingestion, or congenital causes. In some cases, the cause is unknown (idiopathic). Most seizures are brief. If a seizure lasts longer than 5 min, anticonvulsant medications will need to be administered (Fig. 2.6).

History	Seizure onset
	Prior seizures
	Intercurrent illness, fever
	Medications (type, dose, route, compliance, recent changes) and ingestion history
	Trauma (especially head trauma)
Immediate	Place patient in supine position
Assessment	Assess airway, neurological status, temperature, glucose level, injury
Management	Prepare to secure airway. Anticipate need for assisted ventilation at any time
	Suction mouth if necessary. Administer oxygen. Attach pulse oximeter
	Recovery position (on side) if vomiting
	Do not use bite block
	Obtain vital signs including pulse oximetry. Reassess airway, breathing, and circulation

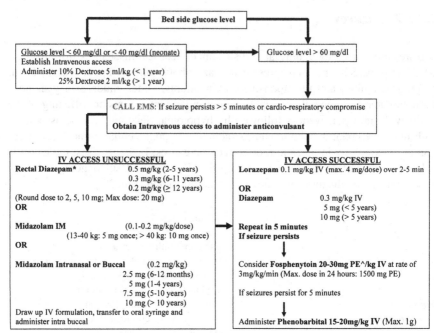

Fig. 2.6   Seizure Protocol

Within the figure:

Bed side glucose level

Glucose level < 60 mg/dl or < 40 mg/dl (neonate)
Establish Intravenous access
Administer 10% Dextrose 5 ml/kg (< 1 year)
              25% Dextrose 2 ml/kg (> 1 year)

Glucose level > 60 mg/dl

CALL EMS: If seizure persists > 5 minutes or cardio-respiratory compromise

Obtain Intravenous access to administer anticonvulsant

IV ACCESS UNSUCCESSFUL
Rectal Diazepam*   0.5 mg/kg (2-5 years)
                             0.3 mg/kg (6-11 years)
                             0.2 mg/kg (≥ 12 years)
(Round dose to 2, 5, 10 mg; Max dose: 20 mg)
OR

Midazolam IM   (0.1-0.2 mg/kg/dose)
              (13-40 kg: 5 mg once; > 40 kg: 10 mg once)
OR

Midazolam Intranasal or Buccal   (0.2 mg/kg)
                             2.5 mg (6-12 months)
                             5 mg (1-4 years)
                             7.5 mg (5-10 years)
                             10 mg (> 10 years)
Draw up IV formulation, transfer to oral syringe and
administer intra buccal

IV ACCESS SUCCESSFUL
Lorazepam 0.1 mg/kg IV (max. 4 mg/dose) over 2-5 min

OR
Diazepam   0.3 mg/kg IV
                             5 mg (< 5 years)
                             10 mg (> 5 years)

Repeat in 5 minutes
If seizure persists

Consider Fosphenytoin 20-30mg PE^/kg IV at rate of
3mg/kg/min (Max. dose in 24 hours: 1500 mg PE)

If seizures persist for 5 minutes

Administer Phenobarbital 15-20mg/kg IV (Max. 1g)

* <2 years: safety/efficacy not established   ^ PE: Phenytoin sodium equivalents

2.8.1.10 Shock and Anaphylaxis

It is a clinical state manifested by inadequate tissue perfusion, resulting in the inability to supply the body with oxygen and nutrients to meet the metabolic demands of the tissues. The signs include those of inadequate perfusion and organ function. Compensated shock is the presence of shock with normal blood pressure (BP).

Most common causes of shock in the pediatric office are hypovolemia (dehydration), sepsis, and anaphylaxis.

Assessment: Tachycardia, weak peripheral and/or central pulses, dyspnea, low BP, skin mottling, increased capillary refill time (>2 s), altered mental status (drowsiness or combativeness), and reduced urine output.

Management: Rapid cardiopulmonary assessment and follow appropriate protocol (Fig. 2.7)

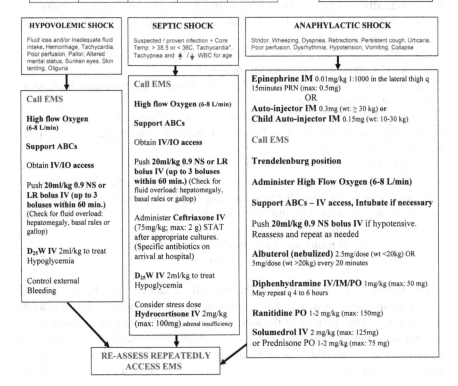

*Upper limit of normal Heart Rates for different temperatures				
	0-23 months	2-5 years	6-12 years	≥ 13 years
< 100F	180	140	130	110
101 F	185	145	135	115
102 F	190	150	140	120
103 F	195	155	145	125
104 F	200	160	150	130
105 F	205	165	155	135

Hypotension (Systolic BP in mmHg)

Term Neonates < 60
Infants (1-10mo) < 70
Child (1-10 y) < 70 + (age x 2)
Children (>10 y) < 90

HYPOVOLEMIC SHOCK

Fluid loss and/or Inadequate fluid intake, Hemorrhage, Tachycardia, Poor perfusion, Pallor, Altered mental status, Sunken eyes, Skin tenting, Oliguria

Call EMS

High flow Oxygen (6-8 L/min)

Support ABCs

Obtain IV/IO access

Push **20ml/kg 0.9 NS or LR bolus IV (up to 3 boluses within 60 min.)** (Check for fluid overload: hepatomegaly, basal rales or gallop)

D₂₅W IV 2ml/kg to treat Hypoglycemia

Control external Bleeding

SEPTIC SHOCK

Suspected / proven infection + Core Temp. > 38.5 or < 36C, Tachycardia*, Tachypnea and ↑ / ↓ WBC for age

Call EMS

High flow Oxygen (6-8 L/min)

Support ABCs

Obtain IV/IO access

Push **20ml/kg 0.9 NS or LR bolus IV (up to 3 boluses within 60 min.)** (Check for fluid overload: hepatomegaly, basal rales or gallop)

Administer **Ceftriaxone IV** (75mg/kg; max: 2 g) STAT after appropriate cultures. (Specific antibiotics on arrival at hospital)

D₂₅W IV 2ml/kg to treat Hypoglycemia

Consider stress dose **Hydrocortisone IV** 2mg/kg (max: 100mg) adrenal insufficiency

ANAPHYLACTIC SHOCK

Stridor, Wheezing, Dyspnea, Retractions, Persistent cough, Urticaria, Poor perfusion, Dysrhythmia, Hypotension, Vomiting, Collapse

Epinephrine IM 0.01mg/kg 1:1000 in the lateral thigh q 15minutes PRN (max: 0.5mg)
OR
Auto-injector IM 0.3mg (wt: ≥ 30 kg) or
Child Auto-injector IM 0.15mg (wt: 10-30 kg)

Call EMS

Trendelenburg position

Administer High Flow Oxygen (6-8 L/min)

Support ABCs – IV access, Intubate if necessary

Push **20ml/kg 0.9 NS bolus IV** if hypotensive. Reassess and repeat as needed

Albuterol (nebulized) 2.5mg/dose (wt <20kg) OR 5mg/dose (wt >20kg) every 20 minutes

Diphenhydramine IV/IM/PO 1mg/kg (max: 50 mg) May repeat q 4 to 6 hours

Ranitidine PO 1-2 mg/kg (max: 150mg)

Solumedrol IV 2 mg/kg (max: 125mg) or Prednisone PO 1-2 mg/kg (max: 75 mg)

RE-ASSESS REPEATEDLY ACCESS EMS

Fig. 2.7 Shock Protocols

2.9 Children with Special Healthcare Needs

2.9.1 Emergency Information Form

Children with multiple health problems and complex case management plans are at risk of receiving suboptimal care in emergency situations. These patients are usually prescribed multiple medications and may be dependent on technologic devices or receive care from multiple specialties. A comprehensive medical history detailing all this information may run into several pages. Accessing and reviewing information from these lengthy medical records is challenging for a treating physician during an emergency. A summary of all the child's conditions, if available, would be very beneficial to the emergency health provider when treating the patient.

Several years ago, the American Academy of Pediatric (AAP) and American College of Emergency Physicians (ACEP) introduced the emergency information form (EIF) (AAP 1999). This was a single-sheet document which summarized the patient's medical history. Unfortunately, this form has not been used widely. Compared to the electronic medical record, the paper-based form is limited in its ability to transfer all the salient history of the patient to the emergency medicine physician. Efforts are underway to prepare an all-inclusive, computerized version of the EIF. The advantages are that it can be regularly updated and can be modified periodically to remain current with changes in health and legal requirements. In addition, these records can be accessed remotely at any time—a feature that is very useful when disasters occur.

The ideal emergency information form for children with special healthcare needs should include the following information:

Identifying Information: Name, birth date, address, parents or guardians, contact information, and emergency contacts

Names of Physicians and Health Providers: A list of the primary-care provider, treating specialist(s), pharmacy and preferred emergency department, and hospital with contact information

Baseline Clinical Condition: All the diagnoses with the most important one first. Baseline physical findings, vital signs, neurological status, whether immune compromised, medications, allergies, baseline laboratory results, advanced directives and if any procedures should be avoided and why.

Immunization Status

List of current ED problems and method of treatment

Disasters most likely to be faced by the patient

The AAP and ACEP recommend that the EIF should be filled by the medical home primary-care physician and incorporate recommendations from the treating specialists. The updating of the form is the responsibility of the medical home doctor and should be done, preferably every six months. End-of-life planning and advance directives should also be included. Electronic health records are being used increasingly in the US (AAP 2010). However, some practices may not have an electronic version of the EIF. The old paper form though inadequate may be manually modified until a computerized EIF standard is developed.

2.9.2 Emergencies

The most common emergencies faced by children with special healthcare needs are as follows:

1. **Tracheostomy complications**: The most important complication is if the tracheostomy tube becomes obstructed (plugged) or gets dislodged. In both situations, the patient will need to have a replacement tracheostomy tube inserted. The caregivers of these patients are instructed to carry with them all the supplies that are essential for changing a tracheostomy tube. This includes a bag–mask ventilation device, suction and oxygen source, replacement cannula, endotracheal tubes of the same and smaller size, scissors, ties, and padding. Additionally, they are educated on how to respond to these emergencies. It is helpful to obtain their information, advice, and assistance in these situations.

Initially, high-flow oxygen should be supplied while rapidly assessing the cardiorespiratory status of the patient with a potentially obstructed tracheostomy tube. Careful suction of the tracheostomy tube should be performed using one to two milliliters of normal saline and the largest size suction cannula on hand. Suction is applied for about 5 s. The child will usually cough when the catheter has gone deep enough. Continue to monitor the child's cardiorespiratory status. If this procedure is unsuccessful, the tracheostomy tube should be changed with the same size tube or one size smaller. With the child laying supine with a towel roll under the neck, an assistant steadies the head and the old tube is removed. This is done by deflating the tube cuff, removing the ties that secure the tube to the neck, and gently pulling out the tube. Lubricate the new tube with the obturator in place. The operator gently inserts the tube into the stoma, pushing posteriorly and inferiorly in an arc. The tube is inserted until the flanges are flush with the neck. The obturator is removed. There should be an improvement in the respiratory status with equal breath sounds heard bilaterally. The tube is secured using the tracheostomy ties and padded to avoid neck irritation. If changing the tracheostomy tube is unsuccessful, the patient may be bagged through the mouth (unless the child has tracheal diversion surgery) or the stoma.

2. **Gastrostomy complications**: These include blocked or dislodged tubes or skin irritation due to leaking of stomach contents around the tube.
   (a) If the enterostomy tube is blocked, one can attempt to relieve the obstruction by flushing the tube with warm water or a carbonated beverage.
   (b) A dislodged gastrostomy tube should be replaced as soon as possible since the fistula will rapidly close if the tube remains out for any length of time. If the tract is well formed and long-standing (>8 weeks after surgery) and a replacement tube is unavailable, a Foley catheter may

be placed to maintain the patency of the tract. The patient should be promptly referred to the emergency department for insertion of a replacement tube.

(c) Skin irritation around the fistula opening can be treated with frequent changes in saline-soaked dressings at the site and the application of barrier creams. Sometimes the tube may have to be attached a bit tighter or replaced. Referral to the surgeon or intervention radiologist is advised.

3. **Respiratory distress**: This should be assessed like any other patients with respiratory distress. They should receive oxygen if hypoxic and bronchodilators if there is bronchospasm. Such patients should be referred to the emergency department.

4. **Diarrhea/dehydration**: Patients should be assessed for dehydration and receive fluid replacement if dehydrated. If they are in circulatory shock due to severe dehydration, they should be stabilized and transferred to the emergency department. These patients are placed on oxygen and resuscitated with fluids administered either intravenously or by intra-osseous route. (see shock protocol).

5. **Prolonged seizures**: These patients should have a rapid cardiorespiratory assessment. Seizure control and stabilization of cardio-respiratory status are the most important goals. (see seizure protocol).

2.10 Psychosocial Emergencies

Eileen R. Giardino, RN, PhD, FNP-BC, Michelle A. Lyn, MD and Angelo P. Giardino, MD, PhD

Pediatric clinicians in the office-based setting may confront a number of psychosocial situations which require rapid responses to ensure the safety of the child or adolescent and in the case of child maltreatment, for example, to comply with the legally mandated reporting responsibility present in all 50 states of the United States. This section describes psychosocial emergencies that include child physical abuse, child sexual abuse, exposure to intimate partner violence, and the risk for suicide.

1. **Child Physical Abuse**:

A basic definition of child physical abuse is when a caregiver causes injury to a child. The typical presentation for child physical abuse in a physician's office is a child who presents with an injury. The physician must be aware of injury patterns that might indicate the possibility of child physical abuse because the caregiver may provide an incomplete or misleading history, and most injuries will not be pathognomonic for child abuse. In 2010, at least 118,700 children were known to have been physically abused by a caregiver and sadly, at least 1,700 children died as a result of that abuse. *Identification*:

Presentations that should raise suspicion for physical abuse include the following:

- History that is inconsistent or not plausible with the physical examination
- History of no trauma but evidence of injury on physical examination (i.e., magical injury)
- History of self-inflicted trauma that is incompatible with child's developmental level
- Evolving history of injury that changes over time
- Inordinate delay in seeking medical treatment
- Serious injury is blamed on young sibling or playmate

Response:

As in all serious injuries, the first response by the healthcare professional should be immediate attention to assessment of stability and managing of airway and circulation. When the child is stable, a thorough healthcare evaluation is completed and includes a history, physical examination, appropriate imaging, and laboratory studies. Also, the clinician considers all differential diagnoses of medical conditions along with the possibility of child physical abuse. When child physical abuse is suspected during the healthcare evaluation, all 50 states require or mandate that a physician or nurse makes a report of that suspicion to appropriate authorities, such as child protective services and/or law enforcement. If the clinical situation is unclear, healthcare professionals likely have access to a regional child abuse team and/or a pediatric emergency department which may be available for an urgent consultation and advice. However, the safety of the child is of paramount importance, and one's mandated reporting responsibility cannot be ignored or delegated to the child abuse expert at a distant location unless careful follow-up occurs to confirm that the child was evaluated in a timely manner. Figure 2.8 provides guidance as to how to respond to the suspicion of child physical abuse.

2. **Child Sexual Abuse**:

Child sexual abuse usually occurs in the context where a more powerful person in a caregiving role involves a developmentally immature child or adolescent in sexual activities for the dominant person's sexual stimulation or gratification. If the abusive person is not in a caregiving role, then this represents child sexual assault rather than abuse. The sexual activities span a wide range of contact and non-contact behaviors including exhibitionism, inappropriate viewing of the child, allowing the child to view inappropriate sexual material, taking sexually related photographs, sexualized kissing, fondling, masturbation, digital or object penetration of the vagina or anus, oral–genital contact, genital–genital contact, and genital–anal contact. Child sexual abuse by its very nature is a betrayal of the child or adolescent's trust in the caregiver and may or may not leave any physical findings or physical injuries. In 2010, at least 63,300 children were known to have been sexually abused.

Identification:

Child sexual abuse may present in a variety of ways in the office setting. The most common presentation involves the evaluation of non-specific behavioral symptoms, such as poor school performance, change in eating or sleeping habits,

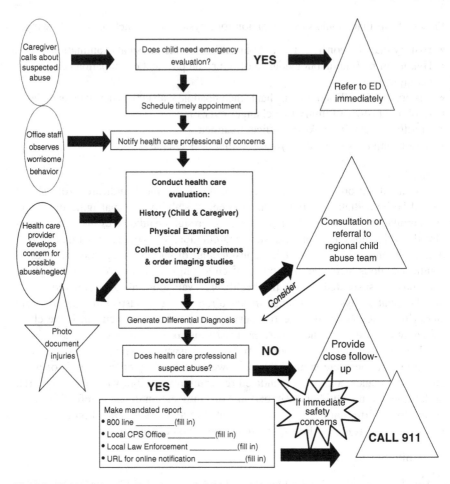

Fig. 2.8 Guidance in reporting suspected child sexual abuse

and/or an unexplained behavior change. Some children purposefully seek out a trusted adult and disclose the inappropriate sexual contact (i.e., makes an outcry). Occasionally, someone in the child's environment raises a concern about possible sexual abuse and alerts those in authority about the concerns and careful questioning by adults in the child's environment which may prompt the child or adolescent to disclose the abuse. In all of these situations, the child or adolescent is vulnerable to the tumult that will ensue once child protective services and law enforcement become involved and conduct their investigation. Consequently, it is essential to pay careful attention to the child's mental health needs during the investigation.

All 50 states of the United States mandate healthcare professionals to report suspected child sexual abuse to child protective services and/or law enforcement. In many communities, child sexual abuse experts may be available for consultation in pediatric emergency departments, child advocacy centers and/or in regional children's hospitals. These resources are valuable in assisting with the evaluation of child sexual abuse. The clinician's mandated responsibility is imperative, and follow-up care is appropriate to ensure that the child is safe and appropriate action is initiated.

Response:

In suspected child sexual abuse, the healthcare evaluation is an essential component to the overall investigation conducted by child protective services/law enforcement. The history-taking process in child sexual abuse is critically important and is defined by an approach that uses non-leading open-ended questions that do not introduce details of a sexual nature unless first raised by the child or adolescent. Once the history is complete, a thorough, head-to-toe physical examination is necessary. The complete physical examination is needed to avoid placing excessive focus on the child's genital region since adults can make the genitals an inappropriate focus of attention. Healthcare professionals should avoid doing the same.

The physical examination is an opportunity to build rapport with the child and to reassure him/her of their wholeness and health despite the abuse. Depending on the symptoms and the circumstances of the case, the collection of laboratory specimens may be necessary to determine the presence of sexually transmitted infections. Depending on the timing of the potential sexual contact, the collection of specimens for a forensic evidence kit might also be indicated. It is important to determine careful differential diagnoses to consider medical diagnoses along with the possibility of child sexual abuse. Mandated reporting must occur when sexual abuse is suspected. Figure 2.8 provides guidance in reporting suspected child sexual abuse.

3.   **Intimate Partner Violence**:

Family violence remains a pervasive problem in our society, and adult caregivers with children may be at risk for being harmed by intimate partners. In families where intimate partner violence exists, the children and adolescents are at increased risk for being physically and/or emotionally harmed. The risk for physical injury is observed in several scenarios: (1) child injured when caught between adults when one is violent toward the other, for example, mother is holding the baby when the violent intimate partner throws and punches at her, and the baby is hit during the attack; (2) child is injured during efforts to protect the caregiver who is being injured by the violent perpetrator; (3) child is targeted for abuse by the violent perpetrator; and finally, (4) excessive discipline of the child by the caregiver who is the victim of violence in order to control the environment in hopes of lessening the risk of violent eruptions of perpetrator's anger which places the child at risk for injury when (e.g., the child's impulsive nature leads to the application of excessive corporal punishment).

The harm to the child may be physical, but emotional harm occurs when a child is exposed to interpersonal violence and its aftermath.

Identification:

Since 1998, the American Academy of Pediatrics has recommended the routine screening of the adult caregivers of pediatric patients for the presence of intimate partner violence in their household. Formal screening approaches are

Fig. 2.9 Radar for pediatrics © 2002 RADAR Pocket Card for Pediatricians developed by The ▶ Institute for Safe Families and the PA Chapter, American Academy of Pediatrics. Philadelphia, PA, 215-843-2046, www.instituteforsafefamilies.org. RADAR acronym developed by the Mass Medical Society. © 1992 Mass Medical Society. Used with permission PDFs with the radar Mneumonic and suitable for reproduction are available free of charge from: http://www.institutef orsafefamilies.org/pdf/healthcare/PedRADARcard.pdf

recommended in order to make it easier to implement screening processes in the office-based setting. Suggested questions used in a pediatric setting include the following:

- How would you characterize your relationship with your partner?
- All couples argue. How do you and your partner handle disagreements or fights?
- Are you in a relationship in which you are being hurt?
- Does your partner ever push, grab, slap, choke, or hit you?
- Does your partner ever force you to have sex or perform sexual acts you did not want to do?
- Are you worried that your partner might hurt your child?

Formal screening tools facilitate the routine screening of adult caregivers of pediatric patients for the presence of intimate partner violence. The radar screening tool is useful to use on a regular basis, which is spelled out in Fig. 2.9.

Response:

Many clinicians who a focused on the care of children are not familiar with the interventions necessary to assist adult victims of intimate partner violence to think through safety planning and address steps to respond to violence and abuse. Clinicians can help patients and caregivers link to community organizations that serve adult victims of intimate partner violence. It is important to know how to assist children and adults with safety planning for those who live in abusive environments. It is essential to establish protocols in the office environment to guide the referral of adult victims of intimate partner violence to community experts who can help those victims deal with the violence in their lives. Knowing available community resources will then help clinicians make appropriate referrals in an efficient manner when the need for one arises. Figure 2.10 is helpful when dealing with a positive screen for intimate partner violence.

4. **Suicide**:

Preventing suicide in those patients at risk for harming themselves remains a high priority for healthcare professionals. A number of risk factors have been identified, and sorting out who is at high risk for attempting suicide and getting them into a system of care that can keep them safe during that mental health crisis is an important part of the office-based response to suicide risk. The Surgeon General's 2012 National Strategy for Suicide Prevention contains several definitions that are important to consider:

Suicide: death caused by self-directed injurious behavior with any intent to die as a result of the behavior

RADAR

FOR PEDIATRICS: A DOMESTIC VIOLENCE INTERVENTION

R = ROUTINELY SCREEN MOTHERS FOR ABUSE

Intervening on behalf of battered women is an active form of preventing child abuse. Victims of violence are very likely to disclose abuse to a health care provider, but only if they are asked about it. Always interview the parent alone if the child is over two years old.

A = ARE YOU BEING HURT?

Ask questions routinely in the course of taking a social history in the context of safety and discipline. "The safety of moms can affect the health and safety of children, so I want to ask you some personal questions." "Because violence is common in so many women's lives, I've begun to ask about it routinely:" "Is there anyone who has physically or sexually hurt you or frightened you?" "Have you ever been hit, kicked, or punched by your partner?" "I notice you have a number of bruises; did someone do this to you?"

IF THE MOTHER ANSWERS "YES", SEE OTHER SIDE FOR RESPONSES AND CONTINUE WITH THE FOLLOWING STEPS:

D = DOCUMENT YOUR FINDINGS

Document in the pediatric chart that RADAR screening was done. Indicate response as "+", "-", or "suspected." Ask Mom if it is safe to document in chart. If yes, use statements such as "the child's mother states she was..." With her permission, include the name of the assailant in your record. "She says her boyfriend, John Smith, struck her..." Note any obvious injuries to the mother. Offer her help in arranging for appropriate medical services.

A = ASSESS SAFETY OF MOTHER AND CHILDREN

Before she leaves the medical setting, find out if it is safe for her and her children to go home. Has there been an increase in frequency or severity of violence? Have there been threats of homicide or suicide? Is there a gun or other weapon present? Have there been threats to children or pets? Are the children currently being abused or in immediate danger?

R = RESPOND, REVIEW OPTIONS & REFER

Know in-house and local resources for referral. If the patient is in imminent danger, find out if there is someone with whom she can stay. Does she need immediate access to a shelter? Offer her the opportunity to use a private phone. If she does not need immediate help, offer information about hotlines and resources in the community (see other side). Offer to write down phone numbers if it is unsafe to take information. Remember that it may be dangerous for her to have these in her possession. Discuss the effects of family violence on children. Do the children need a referral? Make a follow-up appointment to see her and her children and document the options discussed.

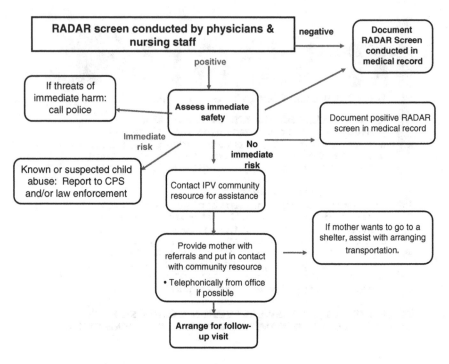

Fig. 2.10 Radar screening

Suicide attempt: a non-fatal, self-directed injurious behavior with any intent to die as a result of the behavior (avoid using term suicide gesture since it appears to minimize the risk)

Suicidal ideation: thoughts of engaging in suicide-related behavior.

Suicidal behaviors: behaviors related to suicide, including preparatory acts, suicide attempts, and deaths.

Each year in the United States, more than 33,000 Americans die as a result of suicide. Approximately 1,500 of these deaths are in teens aged 15 to 19, and in 2009, 4,630 people between 10 and 24 years of age died as a result of suicide. More 9th to 12th graders attempt suicide than actually die from suicide and upward of 16 % of these students reported seriously considering suicide and 13 % actually have created a plan to do so. The CDC reports that each year approximately 157,000 people between 10 and 24 years of age receive medical care in US emergency departments for self-inflicted injuries.

Figure 2.11 displays the percentage of male and female high school students who have considered planned or attempted suicide in 2009:

Identification:

No specific test can identify patients who will commit suicide, but screening for risk factors can identify those at high risk level of acting on those thoughts and plans. Being aware of the risk factors can help the pediatric health professional identify those patients at risk, and certainly, those who have previously attempted suicide as well

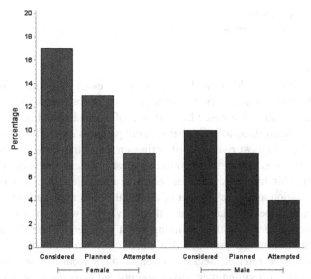

Among high school students in the United States, females were more likely to report having considered, planned, and attempted suicide compared to males (considered suicide: 17.4% versus 10.5%, planned suicide: 13.2% versus 8.6%, and attempted suicide: 8.1% versus 4.6%, respectively) in 2009.

Fig. 2.11 National suicide statistics at a glance. Percent of US high school students reporting, considering, planning, or attempting suicide in the past 12 months, by sex, United States, 2009. *Footnote* *Percentages weighted to be nationally representative

as those who have a well-thought-out plan would be considered at the highest risk. Certain protective factors also have been identified which if present may help mitigate the risk. These are no absolutes however and each case must be considered and the clinician must determine how high the risk is for a given patient and act accordingly with the prevention of suicide in mind. So, patients who express thoughts of suicide and who have the following factors present would be considered at relatively high risk:

- A detailed plan for how to carry out the suicide
- Previous suicide attempt
- Firearms in the household
- Mental illness and/or substance use disorder
- Non-suicidal self-injury
- A friend or family member who has attempted or committed suicide
- Low self-esteem
- A real or anticipated event causing shame, guilt, humiliation, loss of face

Protective factors to consider by the healthcare professional during the healthcare evaluation which may help mitigate the risk in a specific patient include the following (but of course which do not cancel out the risk):

- Family connectedness
- Academic achievement

- School connectedness
- Reduced access to firearms
- Self-esteem

Response:

The response to a child or adolescent who expresses thoughts of suicide and who is therefore at risk for suicide is an urgent matter for everyone involved. The approach taken by an office-based healthcare professional would be based on how high the risk is determined to be in that specific patient's case. Those children and adolescents at the highest risk level of acting on those thoughts are those with a detailed plan and who during the encounter appear hopeless and intent on carrying out their plan. This high-risk situation warrants immediate inpatient hospitalization for stabilization and development of a mental health management plan. Those who do not have a specific plan to harm themselves and who can state clearly that they do not intend to act on their thinking about suicide can be referred urgently to a mental health provider provided that close follow-up is put in place to assure compliance with the referral. Seeking a commitment from the patient about not acting on the idea of harming themselves and instead agreeing to seek help immediately if those thoughts become more pressing is an important part of a contract for safety and is essential in determining risk level; making a contract for safety lowers risk; not making the contract is of great concern and makes the patient high risk. Figure 2.12 lists a flow diagram that helps guide the response to a patient who expresses thoughts of suicide.

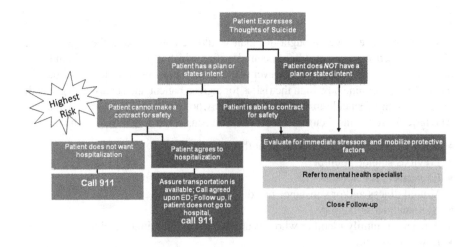

Used/modified with permission
http://reachnola.org/pdfs/suicideriskalgorithm.pdg

Fig. 2.12   Guide when patient expresses thoughts of suicide

2.11 The Primary-Care Pediatrician and Disaster Planning

A disaster is a calamity that affects a large population and generally results in injury, death, and property loss. It overburdens or overwhelms the local response. It can be caused by natural disasters such as hurricanes, tornadoes, earthquakes, fires and blizzards, or man-made conditions such as large transportation-related disasters and terrorist incidents. People may also attempt to evacuate from an imminent threat such as an impending hurricane. All this can lead to physical, mental, and emotional effects on a large number of people. Children, especially those with special healthcare needs, are the most vulnerable. This summary describes the ways in which a community pediatrician can be a resource to his patients and their families in particular and the community in general in times of disaster (AHRQ 2006)

2.11.1 Response to a Disaster

There are four basic phases of response to a disaster: (1) preparedness (including prevention and planning), (2) actual response to the event, (3) mitigation, (4) recovery (short term and long term).

Physicians participate in preparedness and prevention in many different ways, including immunization programs, dietary advice, health education, and safety precautions and planning. As participants in an emergency action plan, physicians need to help formulate ways of preventing incidents from occurring or limiting the consequences from an incident that has already occurred. Pediatricians should be proactive in providing input regarding the unique needs of children during disasters and ensure that children's issues are included in all preparedness activities.

The actual response to the event, mitigation, and the recovery phase is more a responsibility of the first responders, local government, and regional governmental agencies. In the recovery phase, the objective is to return things to normal or near normal as quickly as possible. It involves short- and long-term recovery measures to help vital life support systems return to minimum operating standards. Community-based pediatricians and their staff should try keeping the office running smoothly and provide care to the best of their abilities. The first step is for every staff member to have a personal family emergency plan. Once staff members are assured that they and their family members are safe, they will be better able to focus on their professional duties. Second, every office needs an emergency plan. This plan should include details for handling an emergency, both in the office and in the community.

Items that should be included in an in-office emergency plan include the following:

- Isolation of the patient and family in case of an infection outbreak
- Personal protective equipment for staff
- Backup and safe storage of medical records
- Plans for a secondary office/practice site
- Contact information for local public health authorities
- Phone numbers and instructions for emergency patient transport

Items that should be included in a plan for an emergency in the community include the following:

- Information sheets and hotline telephone numbers;
- Telephone triage protocols;
- Backup staffing schedules.

Office-based physicians may be unsure of their role or feel that they do not have a role in disaster planning or management, yet emergency pediatricians may need to draw on community pediatricians to provide the best possible management of children. The office-based physician may be asked to help hospital-based pediatricians determine which pediatric patients can be discharged or transferred to another hospital. They also will need to triage their own patients who show up at the practice to determine whether they need to go to the hospital or can be safely managed without emergency care. In addition, office-based pediatricians play a critical role in screening children and their family members for medical and psychological distress.

2.11.2 Communicating with Children and Families in Disasters

During a disaster or terrorist event, children and families will receive correct and incorrect information from a multitude of sources, including friends, media, and public officials. A well-educated and available pediatrician who can appropriately respond to numerous and varied questions can be of great service. Families view pediatricians as their expert resource, and most expect pediatricians to be knowledgeable in areas of concern. Providing expert guidance entails both educating families in anticipation of events and responding to questions during and after actual events.

Pediatricians can play a central role in helping families develop a disaster and terrorism preparedness plan. Family preparedness may include training in cardiopulmonary resuscitation, rendezvous points, lists of emergency telephone numbers, and an out-of-state friend or relative with whom all family members can contact after an event to report their whereabouts and conditions. Family members should know the safest place in the home, make special provisions, know community resources, and have a plan to reunite. Medications for chronic illness and resources for children who depend on technological means for survival should be included in the family preparedness plan. Pediatricians can advise parents on the need for a power of attorney, living will, advance directive, and other important legal documents. In addition, pediatricians should advise parents and other family members to:

- Notify utility companies to provide emergency support for technologically dependent family members during a disaster;
- Maintain a supply of medications and equipment in case availability is disrupted during a disaster;
- Know how to obtain additional medications and equipment during times of a disaster;
- Learn how they can assume the role of in-home healthcare providers who may not be available during a disaster;
- Keep an up-to-date emergency information form to provide healthcare workers with the child's medical information in case the regular care provider is unavailable;
- Know backup hospitals/providers in the region in case primary hospital/specialists/providers cannot be used.

2.11.3 Information for Families

In the event of an infection outbreak or bioterrorist attack, one of the most important and challenging roles for the local pediatrician will be providing information to families with children. Public health and medical facilities will be inundated with requests for information and medical evaluation. As a result, these same agencies have prepared communication messages and information sheets that can be shared with families before and during a crisis. Parents will want information that is age-appropriate for their children, as well as suggestions for ways to answer their children's questions. Pediatricians may want to consider accessing some of these materials and having them available before an emergency occurs.

2.11.4 Advocacy

Pediatricians can play a very important and unique role in advocating for the needs of children and families who seldom receive enough attention in disaster planning. Response resources dedicated to pediatric populations remain unavailable or extremely limited for most emergency medical response activities related to disasters, even though victims often include children. To address this shortcoming, it is vitally important that pediatricians and other representatives of special populations take part in local, state, regional, and federal disaster planning to ensure appropriate care for the most vulnerable populations.

2.12 Equipment for Pediatric Office Emergencies

2.12.1 Oropharyngeal Airway

The oropharyngeal airway is a plastic device which provides an air passage and assists in suction of the mouth and airway. It can only be placed in an unconscious patient with an absent gag reflex. The device fits over the back of the tongue and prevents it from flopping back and obstructing the airway. The correct size of an oropharyngeal airway is when its flange abuts against the angle of the mouth and the other end lies against the angle of the mandible. When inserting this airway, first depress the tongue using a tongue depressor and then insert it along the floor of the mouth (Fig. 2.13a, b).

2.12.2 Nasopharyngeal Airway

The nasopharyngeal airway (or "trumpet") is a soft rubber or plastic tube that allows air to flow easily between the nostril and the pharynx. It can be placed in a conscious patient and can relieve upper airway obstruction due to a large tonsils or a large tongue that flops backward as in an obtunded patient. The correct length of a nasopharyngeal airway is approximately the distance from the tip of the nose to the tragus of the ear. First lubricate the airway and then gently insert it along the floor of the nasal cavity. After insertion, it is secured by taping it to the nose (Fig. 2.13c).

2.12.3 Oxygen Therapy

In the clinic, oxygen is usually available for administration to patients from oxygen cylinder. The older oxygen tanks (see Fig. 2.14) require an oxygen flow regulator to be attached to the tank before use. The oxygen flow regulator is attached

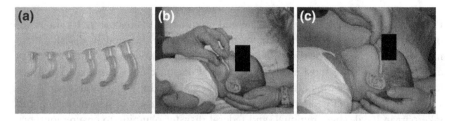

Fig. 2.13 **a–b** Oropharyngeal Airway **c** Nasopharyngeal

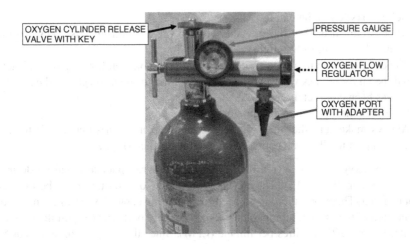

Fig. 2.14 Oxygen cylinder—older version

to the oxygen cylinder release valve. The valve requires a "key" to release oxygen from the cylinder to the oxygen flow regulator. Oxygen is released by turning the key to the left. In addition, a special adapter ("Christmas tree") has to be attached to the oxygen delivery port to allow oxygen tubing to be connected to the patient. The oxygen flow can be regulated from 1/8 to 25 liters per minute (LPM).

Pitfall: There are two places where the oxygen flow can be controlled in the old oxygen tanks: the first is at the oxygen cylinder release valve via the "key" and the second is at the oxygen flow regulator. Before patient use, make sure that both the oxygen release valve and the oxygen flow regulator are open.

After patient use, turn the oxygen cylinder valve off (by turning the key to the right) and "bleed" the residual oxygen in the flow regulator. If the valve is shut off and the residual oxygen not released, the oxygen pressure gage may register a normal pressure. At a future use, if the cylinder valve is not checked to be open (i.e., it is turned off) and the oxygen flow regulator is turned on, there will be a small amount of oxygen released. The user may mistake the oxygen flow to be adequate. In this situation, the oxygen flow will rapidly drop and the patient will not receive adequate oxygen leading to hypoxia. Therefore, before oxygen use, make sure that both the oxygen release valve and the oxygen flow regulator are turned to the open position.

Steps for using oxygen:

1. Open the oxygen cylinder valve by turning the "key" to the left (left—loose; right—tight).
2. Open the oxygen flow regulator and let the oxygen flow at the desired rate to the patient, making sure that the oxygen pressure on the gage is in the acceptable (green) range.

3. Deliver oxygen to the patient.
4. After patient use, shut the oxygen cylinder valve by turning the "key" to the right (left—loose; right—tight).
5. "Bleed" the remaining oxygen out by opening the oxygen flow regulator. There will be an initial hiss which will stop once all the residual oxygen in the regulator has been completely released.
6. Now, turn the oxygen flow regulator off.
7. Always make sure that the cylinder has an adapter ("Christmas tree") for the oxygen port to allow the patient tubing to be attached (Fig. 2.14).

The newer oxygen tanks have a built-in-oxygen flow regulator to release a desired flow of oxygen (Fig. 2.15). The oxygen port allows oxygen tubing to be directly attached to it. Therefore, there is no need for a special adapter ("Christmas tree") for connection of the oxygen tubing to the oxygen delivery port. The oxygen flow can be regulated from 0.25–25 litres per minute (LPM). Since the oxygen pressure is at 50 psi, the oxygen port can also be connected directly to a ventilator during transport of an unstable patient. The colour of the oxygen cylinder is silver with a green top and a green handle. If the handle is colored orange, the oxygen clinder is MRI compatible.

2.12.4 Oxygen Mask

A non-rebreathing oxygen mask (see Figs. 2.16) should be used when the patient needs to be administered the maximum possible oxygen for hypoxia. Connect the tubing to an oxygen tank and set the oxygen flow to 10–15 L/min. Then, depress the small rubber valve at the top of the bag to inflate the bag so that it can serve as an oxygen reservoir. Then, apply the oxygen mask to the patient. Simple face

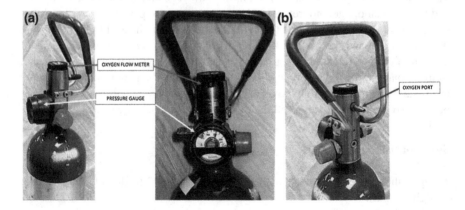

Fig. 2.15 **a** Oxygen cylinder (newer version) flow meter and pressure gauge. **b** oxygen cylinder (newer version) oxygen port

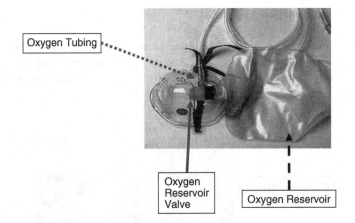

Oxygen Tubing

Oxygen
Reservoir
Valve

Oxygen Reservoir

Fig. 2.16 Non-rebreather Oxygen mask

masks may be used in patients with mild hypoxia. These are usually at an oxygen flow rate of 5L/min.

2.12.5 Suction Apparatus

2.12.5.1 Manual Suction

In an emergency situation, such as a patient with respiratory distress with copious secretions, a simple bulb syringe is very useful for suctioning the oral cavity. Care must be taken to avoid deeper oropharyngeal suction since it may cause gagging and vagal stimulation (Fig. 2.17).

Fig. 2.17 Bulb syringe

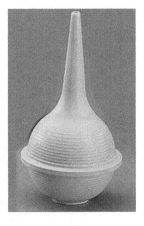

2.12.5.2 Electric Suction Apparatus

The suction apparatus should be a lightweight and powerful portable suction unit with a vacuum regulator and gage. Other supplies that are necessary are a carrying case, 800 cc disposable canister, electricity charger, Yankauer tip, and tubing (Fig. 2.18).

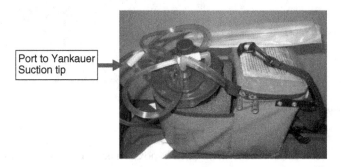

Fig. 2.18 Suction apparatus

2.13   Medications for Pediatric Office Emergencies

Table 2.5   Comparison of pediatric emergency equipment based on rapidity of EMS response

Suggested resuscitation equipment based on EMS response time

	EMS response time >10 min (ex. rural areas)	EMS response time <10 min (ex. urban areas with EMS)
Airway equipment		
Airway	Oropharyngeal airways (infant through adult)	Oropharyngeal airways (infant through adult)
	Nasopharyngeal airways (infant through adult)	Nasopharyngeal airways (infant through adult)
	AMBU-bags and masks (infant, child, and adult)	AMBU-bags and masks (infant, child, and adult)
	Magill forceps (pediatric, adult)	
	Laryngoscope handle(pediatric, adult) with extra batteries	
	Laryngoscope blades (0–2 straight and 2–3 Macintosh)	
	Endotracheal tubes (2.5–8) with stylet (adult, pediatric)	
	End tidal carbon dioxide detector	
Oxygen	Portable oxygen tank(s)	Portable oxygen tank(s)
	Simple mask (pediatric, adult)	Simple mask (pediatric, adult)
	Non-rebreather mask (pediatric, adult)	Non-rebreather mask (pediatric, adult)
Suction	Portable suction machine	Portable suction machine
	Bulb syringe	Bulb syringe
	Tonsil tip (Yankauer) suction catheter with tubing	Tonsil tip (Yankauer) suction catheter with tubing
	Suction catheters (sizes 6, 8, 10, 12)	Suction catheters (sizes 6, 8, 10, 12)
Resuscitation equipment		
AED	Automated external defibrillator (AED)	Automated external defibrillator (AED)
	AED electrode pads (adult, pediatric)	AED electrode pads (adult, pediatric)
Backboard	Cardiac arrest board	Cardiac arrest board

(continued)

Table 2.5 (continued)

Suggested resuscitation equipment based on EMS response time

Length-based color-coded tape (*Broselow*)	Yes	Yes
Fluid resuscitation equipment		
Intra-osseous needles	Sizes 15 and 18	Sizes 15 and 18
Intravenous catheters	Sizes 20, 22, 24	Sizes 20, 22, 24
Intravenous start kit	Yes	Yes
IV tubing and buretrol	Yes	Yes
Venous access supplies	Armboards (2 × 4, 2 × 9); sterile dressing materials (tape, 2 × 2 gauze, 4 × 4 gauze, 2″ gauze wrap)	Armboards (2 × 4, 2 × 9); sterile dressing materials (tape, 2 × 2 gauze, 4 × 4 gauze, 2″ gauze wrap)
Other equipments		
Pulse oximeter, glucometer	Yes	Yes
Nebulizer and MDI spacer	Yes	Yes
BP machine	Yes	Yes
Cervical spine collar	Yes	No

Preparation for Emergencies in the Offices of Pediatricians and Pediatric Primary Care Providers. (2007) Committee on Pediatric Emergency Medicine American Academy of Pediatrics. *Pediatrics*, 120: 200–212 (Tables 2.5 and 2.6)

Table 2.6 Comparison of pediatric emergency medications based on rapidity of EMS response

Suggested emergency medications based on EMS response time	
EMS response time >10 min (ex. rural areas)	EMS response time <10 min (ex. urban areas with EMS)
DRUGS	
Ceftriaxone 1-gram vial	Ceftriaxone 1-gram vial
Dexamethasone (4 mg/ml) 5 ml vial	Dexamethasone (4 mg/ml) 5 ml vial
Prednisolone (15 mg/5 ml) PO	Prednisolone (15 mg/5 ml) PO
Dextrose 25 % (250 mg/ml) 10 ml syringe	Dextrose 25 % (250 mg/ml) 10 ml syringe
Dextrose 50 % (500 mg/ml) 50 ml vial	Dextrose 50 % (500 mg/ml) 50 ml vial
Diazepam (graduated diazepam rectal dispensing mechanisms are permissible as long as the full range of dosing can be achieved)	Diazepam (graduated diazepam rectal dispensing mechanisms are permissible as long as the full range of dosing can be achieved)
Diazepam 2.5 mg rectal suppository	Diazepam 2.5 mg rectal suppository
Diazepam 10 mg rectal suppository OR	Diazepam 10 mg rectal suppository OR
Diazepam (5 mg/ml) injectable vial	Diazepam (5 mg/ml) injectable vial
Lorazepam (2 mg/ml) injectable vial	
Diphenhydramine (50 mg/ml) 1 ml vial	Diphenhydramine (50 mg/ml) 1 ml vial
Epinephrine 1: 10,000 (0.1 mg/1 ml) syringe	Epinephrine 1: 10,000 (0.1 mg/1 ml) syringe
Epinephrine 1: 1000 (1 mg/1 ml) ampoule	Epinephrine 1: 1000 (1 mg/1 ml) ampoule
EpiPen Jr 1:2000 (0.15 mg/0.3 ml)	EpiPen Jr 1:2000 (0.15 mg/0.3 ml)
EpiPen 1:1000 (0.3 mg/0.3 ml)	EpiPen 1:1000 (0.3 mg/0.3 ml)
Normal saline 500 ml bag	Normal saline 500 ml bag
Albuterol for inhalation	Albuterol for inhalation
Activated charcoal	
Sodium bicarbonate (4.2 %)	
Naloxone (0.4 mg/ml)	
Atropine sulfate (0.1 mg/ml)	

Preparation for Emergencies in the Offices of Pediatricians and Pediatric Primary Care Providers. (2007) Committee on Pediatric Emergency Medicine American Academy of Pediatrics. *Pediatrics*, 120: 200–212.

Table 2.7 Emergency medication use in pediatric office emergencies

Medication	Indication	Dosage	Special Considerations
Albuterol	Asthma exacerbation, bronchospasm	*Intermittent aerosol:* 2.5–5 mg diluted in 2–3 ml saline. Administer every 20 min for 3 doses followed by 0.15–0.3 mg/kg up to 10 mg every 1–4 h as needed	Oxygen may be used for nebulization if the patient is also hypoxic
		Metered dose inhaler with spacer: (90 mcg/ puff) 4–8 puffs every 15–20 min for 3 doses. Repeat every 1–4 h as needed	Causes tachycardia, jitteriness, and hypoka- lemia with prolonged aerosol treatments
Sodium bicarbonate	Metabolic acidosis, hyperkalemia, tricyclic antidepressant toxicity	*IV/IO:* 1–2 mEq/kg given slowly	Routine initial use in cardiac arrest is not advised. Administer if documented meta- bolic acidosis and patient is ventilated effectively
Charcoal, activated	Acute ingestion of toxic agent within one hour of presentation	*PO/Nasogastric tube:* 1 g/kg	*Contraindications:* Ingestion of iron, toxic alcohols, caustic agents, lithium
	Call poison center 800-222-1222 before use		*Caution* In obtunded patient who is an aspira- tion risk—may administer after the airway is secured with cuffed endotracheal tube and benefits outweigh risks
Ceftriaxone	Antibiotic	*IM/IV:* 75 mg/kg	
Dexamethasone	Croup	*PO, IM, or IV:* 0.6 mg/kg (max. dose 10 mg)	May use parenteral preparation by oral route
Diazepam	Status epilepticus	*Rectal:* 0.5 mg/kg (2–5 years)	*Caution:* IM route causes tissue necrosis
		0.3 mg/kg (6–11 years)	
		0.2 mg/kg (≥12 years)	
		(Round dose to 2, 5, 10 mg; max. dose: 20 mg)	
		IV: 0.3 mg/kg IV administer slowly	
		5 mg (<5 years)	
		10 mg (>5 years)	May cause apnea

(continued)

Table 2.7 (continued)

Medication	Indication	Dosage	Special Considerations
Dextrose	Hypoglycemia	*IV:* 10 % dextrose: 5 ml/kg (<1 year) 25 % dextrose: 2 ml/kg (>1 year) *PO:* Orange juice 2–4 oz	Care against IV extravasation
Diphenhydramine	Allergic reaction, dystonia	*PO/IV/IM:* 1 mg/kg (max. 50 mg)	Causes sedation. Do not administer rapid IV
Epinephrine	Cardiac pulmonary resuscitation	*IV:* 0.01 mg/kg of 1 : 10,000 solution (max. 1 mg) repeated every 3–5 min	
Epinephrine	Anaphylaxis	*IM:* 0.01 mg/kg of 1:1,000 solution (max. 0.3–0.5 mg)	
Epinephrine	Croup	*Inhalation:* 2.25 % soln. of racemic epinephrine: 0.5 ml	Causes tachycardia
Lorazepam	Status epilepticus	*IV:* 0.1 mg/kg (max. 4 mg/dose) over 2–5 min	Store in refrigerator. May cause apnea
Midazolam	Status epilepticus	*IM:* 0.1–0.2 mg/kg/dose (13–40 kg: 5 mg once; >40 kg: 10 mg once) *Buccal/Intranasal:* 0.2 mg/kg 2.5 mg (6–12 months) 5 mg (1–4 years) 7.5 mg (5–10 years) 10 mg (>10 years)	Draw up IV formulation, transfer to oral syringe, and administer by intra-buccal route May cause apnea
Prednisolone	Acute asthma attack	*PO:* 2 mg/kg (max. 60 mg)	May cause vomiting

References

A) Systems and Priorities

Flores, G., & Weinstock, D. J. (1996). The preparedness of pediatricians for emergencies in the office: what is broken, should we care, and how can we fix it? *Archives of Pediatrics and Adolescent Medicine, 150*(3), 249–256.

Walsh-Kelly, C. M., Bergholte, J., Erschen, M. J., & Melzer-Lange, M. (2004). Office preparedness for pediatric emergencies: baseline preparedness and the impact of guideline distribution. *Pediatric Emergency Care, 20*(5), 289–294.

Shetty, A. K., Hutchinson, S. W., Mangat, R., & Peck, G. Q. (1998). Preparedness of practicing pediatricians in Louisiana to manage emergencies. *Southern Medical Journal, 91*(8), 745–748.

Santillanes, G., Gausche-Hill, M., & Sosa, B. (2006). Preparedness of selected pediatric offices to respond to critical emergencies in children. *Pediatric Emergency Care, 22*(11), 694–698.

Schmitt, B. D. (2010). Pediatric telephone protocols: office version (13th ed.). IL: American Academy of Pediatrics Elk Grove Village.

B) Protocols for Common Pediatric Office Emergencies Asthma

National Heart, Lung, and Blood Institute, National Asthma Education and Prevention Program, Expert Panel Report 3: Guidelines for the Diagnosis and Management of Asthma, Full Report, U.S. Department of Health and Human Services, National Institutes of Health, 2007.

Murphy, K. R., Hopp, R. J., Kittelson, E. B., Hansen, G., Windle, M. L., & Walburn, J. N. (2006). Life-threatening asthma and anaphylaxis in schools: a treatment model for school-based programs. *Annals of Allergy, Asthma and Immunology, 96*(3), 398–405.

Clinical Guidelines. (2012). Asthma guideline evidence-based outcome center—Texas Children's Hospital, Houston, Texas. Accessed 18 Sept 2012.

Castro-Rodriguez, J. A., & Rodrigo, G. J. (2004). Beta-agonists through metered-dose inhaler with valved holding chamber versus nebulizer for acute exacerbation of wheezing or asthma in children under 5 years of age: a systematic review with meta-analysis. *Journal of Pediatrics, 145*(2), 172–177.

Rowe, B. H., Spooner, C. H., Ducharme, F. M., Bretzlaff, J. A. & Bota, G. W. (2007). Corticosteroids for preventing relapse following acute exacerbations of asthma. *Cochrane Database of Systematic Reviews*, Issue 3. Art. No.: CD0001 95. doi:10.1002/14651858. CD000195.pub2.

Blunt Head Trauma

Kuppermann, N., Holmes, J. F., Dayan, P. S., et al. (2009). Identification of children at very low risk of clinically-important brain injuries after head trauma: a prospective cohort study. *The Lancet, 374*(9696), 1160–1170.

Bronchiolitis

Diagnosis and Management of Bronchiolitis. (2006). American academy of pediatrics subcommittee on diagnosis and management of bronchiolitis. *Pediatrics, 118*(4), 1774–1793.

Bronchiolitis Guideline Team, Cincinnati Children's Hospital Medical Center. (2012). Evidence based clinical practice guideline for medical management of bronchiolitis in infants 1 year of age or less presenting with a first time episode. Guideline 1, pp. 1–13. http://www.cincinnatichildrens.org/service/j/anderson-center/evidence-based-care/bronchiolitis/. Accessed 23 Sept 2012.

Viswanathan, M., King, V., & Bordley, C. (2003). Management of bronchiolitis in infants and children. Evidence report/Technology assessment no. 69. AHRQ Publication No. 03-E014. Rockville, MD: U.S. Department of Health and Human Services, Agency for Healthcare Research and Quality.

Mansback, J. M., Clark, S., Christopher, N. C., LoVecchio, R., Kunz, S., Acholonu, U., et al. (2008). Prospective multicenter study of bronchiolitis: predicting safe discharges from the emergency department. *Pediatrics, 121*(4), 680–688.

Levine, D. A., Platt, S. L., Dayan, P. S., Macias, C. G., Zorc, J. J., Krief, W., et al. (2004). Risk of serious bacterial infection in young febrile infants with respiratory syncytial virus infections. *Pediatrics, 113*(6), 1728–1734.

Cardiac Arrest

Kleinman, M. E., Chameides, L., Schexnayder, S. M., Samson, R. A., Hazinski, M. F., Atkins, D. L., et al. (2010a). Part 14: pediatric advanced life support: 2010 American heart association guidelines for cardiopulmonary resuscitation and emergency cardiovascular care. *Circulation, 122*(3), S876–S908.

Kleinman, M. E., Chameides, L., Schexnayder, S. M., et al. (2010b). Special report—Pediatric advanced life support: 2010 American heart association guidelines for cardiopulmonary resuscitation and emergency cardiovascular care. *Pediatrics, 126*(5), e1361–1399.

Choking (Infant and Child)

Pediatric Basic Life Support (2000) Resuscitation, 46, 326–329.

Croup

Bjornson, C., Russell, K. F., Vandermeer, B., Durec, T., Klassen, T.P., Johnson, D.W. (2011). Nebulized epinephrine for croup in children. *Cochrane Database of Systematic Reviews*, (2):CD006619.

Russell, K. F., Liang, Y., O'Gorman, K., Johnson, D. W., Klassen, T. P. (2011). Glucocorticoids for croup. *Cochrane Database of Systematic Reviews*, (1):CD001955.

Scolnik, D., Coates, A. L., Stephens, D., Da Silva, Z., Lavine, E., & Schuh, S. (2006). Controlled delivery of high vs low humidity vs mist therapy for croup in emergency departments: a randomized controlled trial. *JAMA: The Journal of the American Medical Association., 295*(11), 1274–1280.

Moore, M., Little, P. (2011). WITHDRAWN: Humidified air inhalation for treating croup. *Cochrane Database of Systematic Reviews*, (6):CD002870.

Diabetic Ketoacidosis

Glaser, N., Barnett, P., McCaslin, I., Nelson, D., Trainor, J., Louie, J., et al. (2001). Risk factors for cerebral edema in children with diabetic ketoacidosis. *New England Journal of Medicine, 344*(4), 264–269.

Lawrence, S. E., Cummings, E. A., Gaboury, I., & Daneman, D. (2005). Population-based study of incidence and risk factors for cerebral edema in pediatric diabetic ketoacidosis. *Journal of Pediatrics, 146*(5), 688–692.

Marcin, J. P., Glaser, N., Barnett, P., McCaslin, I., Nelson, D., Trainor, J., et al. (2002). Factors associated with adverse outcomes in children with diabetic ketoacidosis-related cerebral edema. *Journal of Pediatrics, 141*(6), 793–797.

Wolfsdorf, J., Glaser, N., & Sperling, M. A. (2006). Diabetic ketoacidosis in infants, children, and adolescents: A consensus statement from the American Diabetes Association. *Diabetes Care, 29*(5), 1150–1159.

Clinical Guidelines. (2012). Diabetic Ketoacidosis guideline. Evidence-based outcome center— Texas Children's Hospital, Houston. Accessed 18 Sept 2012.

Seizures

Initial management of seizures (Status Epilepticus) Clinical guideline Evidence-based Outcome Center—Texas Children's Hospital, Houston. Accessed 12 Sept 2012.

Vilke, G. M., Castillo, E. M., Ray, L. U., Murrin, P., & Chan, T. C. (2005). Evaluation of pediatric glucose monitoring and hypoglycemic therapy in the field. *Pediatric Emergency Care, 21*(1), 1–5.

Kumar, G., Sng, B. L., & Kumar, S. (2004). Correlation of capillary and venous blood glucometry with laboratory determination. *Prehospital Emergency Care, 8*(4), 378–383.

Chin, R. F. M., Verhulst, L., Neville, B. G. R., Peters, M. J., & Scott, R. C. (2004). Inappropriate emergency management of status epilepticus in children contributes to need for intensive care. *Journal of Neurology, Neurosurgery and Psychiatry, 75*(11), 1584–1588.

Chin, R. F. M., Neville, B. G. R., Peckham, C., Wade, A., Bedford, H., & Scott, R. C. (2008). Treatment of community-onset, childhood convulsive status epilepticus: a prospective, population-based study. *The Lancet Neurology, 7*(8), 696–703.

McIntyre, J., Robertson, S., Norris, E., Appleton, R., Whitehouse, W. P., Phillips, B., et al. (2005). Safety and efficacy of buccal midazolam versus rectal diazepam for emergency treatment of seizures in children: a randomized controlled trial. *Lancet, 366*(9481), 205–210.

Mpimbaza, A., Ndeezi, G., Staedke, S., Rosenthal, P. J., & Byarugaba, J. (2008). Comparison of buccal midazolam with rectal diazepam in the treatment of prolonged seizures in Ugandan children: a randomized clinical trial. *Pediatrics, 121*(1), e58–64.

Baysun, S., Aydin, O. F., Atmaca, E., & Gurer, Y. K. Y. (2005). A comparison of buccal midazolam and rectal diazepam for the acute treatment of seizures. *Clinical Pediatrics, 44*(9), 771–776.

Bhattacharyya, M., Kalra, V., & Gulati, S. (2006). Intranasal midazolam vs. rectal diazepam in acute childhood seizures. *Pediatric Neurology, 34*(5), 355–359.

Fisgin, T., Gurer, Y., Tezic, T., Senbil, N., Zorlu, P., Okuyaz, C., et al. (2002). Effects of intranasal midazolam and rectal diazepam on acute convulsions in children: prospective randomized study. *Journal of Child Neurology, 17*(2), 123–126.

Prasad, K., Al-Roomi, K., Krishnan, P. R., Sequeira, R. (2005). Anticonvulsant therapy for status epilepticus. *Cochrane Database of Systematic Reviews* 2005, Issue 4. Art. No.: CD003723. doi:10.1002/14651858.CD003723.pub2.

Appleton, R., Macleod, S., Martland, T. (2008). Drug management for acute tonic-clonic convulsions including convulsive status epilepticus in children. *Cochrane Database of Systematic Reviews* 2008, Issue 3. Art. No.: CD001905. doi:10.1002/14651858.CD001905.pub2.

Silbergleit, R., Durkalski, V., Lowenstein, D., Conwit, R., Pancioli, A., Palesch, Y., Barsan, W, NETT Investigators. (2012). Intramuscular versus intravenous therapy for prehospital status epilepticus. *New England Journal of Medicine 366*(7), 591–600.

Shock and Anaphylaxis

Goldstein, B., Giroir, B., & Randolph, A. (2005). International consensus conference on pediatric sepsis international pediatric sepsis consensus conference: definitions for sepsis and organ dysfunction in pediatrics. *Pediatric Critical Care Medicine, 6*(1), 2–8.

Han, Y. Y., Carcillo, J. A., Dragotta, M. A., Bills, D. M., Watson, R. S., Mark, E., et al. (2003). Early reversal of pediatric-neonatal septic shock by community physicians is associated with improved outcome. *Pediatrics, 112,* 793–799.

Carcillo, J. A., & Fields, A. I. (2002). Clinical practice parameters for hemodynamic support of pediatric and neonatal patients in septic shock. *Critical Care Medicine, 30,* 1365–1378.

Dellinger, R. P., Levy, M. M., Carlet, J. M., et al. (2008). Surviving sepsis campaign: international guidelines for management of severe sepsis and septic shock. *Critical Care Medicine, 36*(1), 296–327.

Sampson, H. A., Muñoz-Furlong, A., Campbell, R. L., et al. (2006). Second symposium on the definition and management of anaphylaxis: summary report—second national institute of allergy and infectious disease/food allergy and anaphylaxis network symposium. *Journal of Allergy and Clinical Immunology, 117*(2), 391–397.

Scott, H., Sicherer, F., Estelle, R. & The Section on Allergy and Immunology American Academy of Pediatrics. (2007). Self-injectable epinephrine for first-aid management of anaphylaxis. *Pediatrics 119,* 638–646.

Sampson, H. A. (2003). Anaphylaxis and emergency treatment. *Pediatrics, 111,* 1601–1608.

Special Situations

Emergency Preparedness for Children with Special Health Care Needs. (1999). Committee on pediatric emergency medicine American academy of pediatrics. *Pediatrics, 104*(4), e53.

Policy Statement Emergency Information Forms and Emergency Preparedness for Children with Special Health Care (2010) Needs American Academy of Pediatrics, Committee on Pediatric Emergency Medicine and Council on Clinical Information Technology, American College of Emergency Physicians, Pediatric Emergency Medicine Committee Pediatrics, 125, 829–837.

Pediatric Terrorism and Disaster Preparedness: A Resource for Pediatricians (2006) Summary AHRQ Publication No. 06(07)-0056-1 Rockville, MD: Agency for Healthcare Research and Quality. September 2006.

Bair-Merritt, M. H., & Fein, J. A. (2010). Intimate partner violence and child abuse. In A. P. Giardino & E. R. Giardino (Eds.), *Intimate partner violence: a resource for professionals working with children and families.* St. Louis: STM Learning.

Giardino, A. P., & Lyn, M. A. (2009). The problem. In M. A. Finkel & A. P. Giardino (Eds.), *Medical evaluation of child sexual abuse: a practical guide* (3rd ed.). Elk Grove Village: American Academy of Pediatrics.

Giardino, A. P., Lyn, M. A., & Giardino, E. R. (2010). Introduction: child abuse and neglect. In A. P. Giardino, M. A. Lyn, & E. R. Giardino (Eds.), *A practical guide to the evaluation of child physical abuse and neglect* (2nd ed.). New York: Springer Publishing.

National Center for the Prevention of Youth Suicide. Youth Suicide Behavior Fact Sheet. http://www.suicidology.org/c/document_library/get_file?folderId=232&name=DLFE-335.pdf REACH NOLA. Community and Academic Partnerships. http://reachnola.org/pdfs/suicideriskalgorithm.pdf.

Shain, B. N. (2007). Suicide and suicide attempts in adolescents. *Pediatrics, 120,* 669.

Tscholl, J. J., & Scribano, P. V. (2010). Intimate partner violence. In A. P. Giardino, M. A. Lyn, & E. R. Giardino (Eds.), *A practical guide to the evaluation of child physical abuse and neglect* (2nd ed.). New York: Springer Publishing.

U.S. Department of Health and Human Services, Administration for Children and Families, Administration on Children, Youth and Families, Children's Bureau. (2011). Child Maltreatment 2010. Available from http://www.acf.hhs.gov/programs/cb/stats_research/index.htm#can.

U.S. Centers for Disease Control and Prevention. National Suicide Statistics at a Glance. http://www.cdc.gov/ViolencePrevention/suicide/statistics/youth_risk.html.

U.S. Department of Health and Human Services (HHS) Office of the Surgeon General and National Alliance for Suicide Prevention. *2012 National Strategy for Suicide Prevention: Goals and Objectives for Action*. Washington: HHS, Sept 2012.

Chapter 3
Education of Providers in Pediatric Office Emergency Preparedness

In this chapter, a number of educational tools and teaching materials are provided for use in the training of office staff, as they prepare for the mock code scenarios. In sequence, the materials appear as follows:

1. airway maneuvers,
2. intra-osseous access,
3. automated external defibrillator (AED),
4. life support course descriptions,
5. mock code process,
6. sample mock code scenario,
7. mock code scripts,
   a. reactive airway disease/pneumonia and
   b. active seizures
8. mock code evaluation form,
9. sample test for training evaluation, and
10. office emergency preparedness education program: practitioner needs assessment survey.

Electronic Supplementary Material
The online version of this chapter (doi:10.1007/978-1-4614-6904-9_3) contains supplementary material, which is available to authorized users.

3.1 Airway Maneuvers (Fig. 3.1a–f)

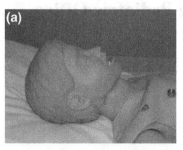

NORMAL POSITION OF HEAD

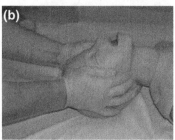

HEAD TILT AND JAW THRUST

The head is tilted posteriorly and the angles of the mandible are pushed anteriorly to open the airway

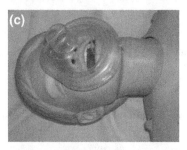

CORRECT SIZE - OXYGEN MASK

The top of the mask should fit on the bridge of the nose and the bottom of the mask should rest just above the chin. There should be a good seal obtained with the face

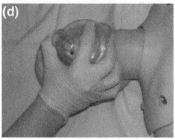

HOLDING OXYGEN MASK BY "E-C" CLAMP TECHNIQUE

The thumb and index finger "C" grasp the oxygen mask and the 3rd, 4th and 5th fingers "E" grasp the mandible to maintain firm contact of the mask with the face

Fig. 3.1 a–f Airway maneuvers

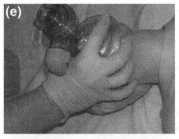

**HOLDING OXYGEN MASK BY
"E-C" CLAMP TECHNIQUE
WITH HEAD TILT**

The same as above but with the head
tilted posteriorly to facilitate ventilation

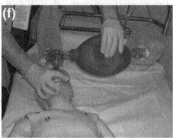

**BAG & MASK VENTILATION
WITH "E-C" CLAMP TECHNIQUE**

One hand holds the oxygen mask by the
"E-C" technique and tilts the head. The
other hand compresses the Ambu bag
which is connected to the mask and an
oxygen source. Ensure that is easy to
compress the Ambu bag and there is
good chest expansion when it is
compressed

Fig. 3.1

3.2 IntraOsseous (IO) Access

Indications: Intraosseous (IO) access is indicated in a patient with cardiopulmonary arrest or circulatory shock where immediate vascular access is required and
attempts at intravenous access have been unsuccessful for 90 s (see Fig. 3.2a–e).

3.2.1 Sites

1. Antero-medial proximal tibia, one finger breadth inferior and medial to the tib-
   ial tuberosity (children under 4 years of age)
2. Area one cm proximal to the medial malleolus, halfway between the anterior
   and posterior borders (children above 4 years of age)
3. Other sites: Distal femur (midline, above the femoral condyles) and anterior–
   superior iliac spine

3.2.2 Contraindications

1. Fracture in the same extremity bone where IO access is planned
2. Previous insertion attempt in the same extremity bone that entered the bone
   marrow
3. Infection overlying the bone
4. Osteogenesis imperfecta

3.2.3 Method

Restrain the patient and isolate the extremity

Use sterile precautions and clean and prepare the area using chlorhexidine scrub if time permits

Locate and mark out the area for insertion

Inject local anesthetic (1 % lidocaine) into the overlying skin and periosteum at the point of IO insertion if the patient is conscious

Place the IO needle hub in the palm and hold the needle with the thumb and index finger (Fig. 3.2d)

Using a steady, rotational back and forth "screwing" technique, insert the IO needle into the bone perpendicular to its long axis angled away from the joint. Continue until a "give" occurs

Confirmation of correct placement of an IO needle: (1) the needle is able to stay erect by itself, (2) bone marrow can be aspirated, and (3) fluids can be administered easily without extravasation into the soft tissues

Holding the winged hub of the IO needle securely and without moving it any further, unscrew the cap from the top of the needle

Remove the needle stylet and attach a 10 ml syringe to the needle

Aspirate the bone marrow contents. You may send this for tests (glucose, culture, etc.)

Connect extension tubing from the needle to a three-way stopcock (Fig. 3.2e)

Attach a 500–1000 ml bag of normal saline to intravenous tubing and attach the tubing to one port of the three-way stopcock

Attach a 20 ml syringe to the other port of the three-way stopcock

Alternately, aspirate 20 ml normal saline from the saline bag and then turn the stopcock to infuse the saline into the bone marrow

Ensure that the fluid flows easily and that there is no soft tissue swelling (If swelling occurs, the IO is improperly placed and another site needs to be accessed)

Secure the IO assembly to the patient, by grasping the needle with a plastic clamp, applying gauze dressing around the assembly and then taping it to the patient

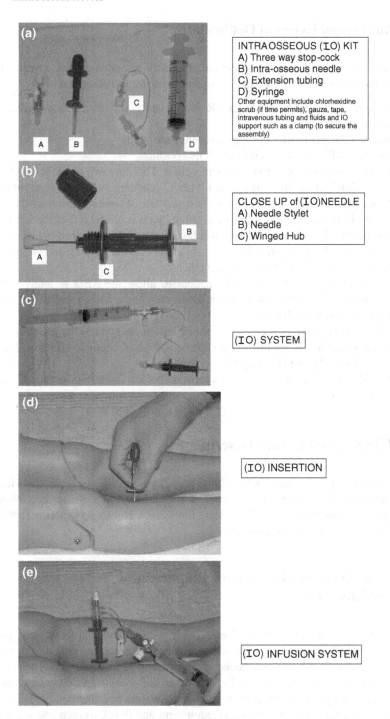

Fig. 3.2 a Intraosseous access kit. **b** Intraosseous access needle. **c** Intraosseous access—IO system. **d** Intraosseous access—needle insertion. **e** Intraosseous—infusion

3.3 Automated External Defibrillator

Providers may be called upon to use an AED during sudden cardiac arrest. The steps in the use of an AED for a patient in cardiac arrest are described below:

1. Begin chest compressions and CPR immediately and dispatch someone to obtain the AED
2. Continue CPR per basic life support recommendations
3. When the AED arrives, turn it to the "ON" position
4. Attach the two chest pads to the patient's chest. There are two sizes for the chest pads: "Infant" (children < 10 kg) and "Adult" (children > 10 kg). The "infant" pads are placed, one on the anterior chest just left of sternum and the other on the back. In the older child, one of the "adult" pads is placed left of the left nipple at the anterior axillary line and over the heart and the other pad is placed on the right infraclavicular area. The pads should not be overlapping and should be separated from each other by at least 3 cm.
5. Clear all providers away from the patient to allow the AED to analyze the heart rhythm. The AED will interpret the rhythm and a voice prompt will state whether a "shock is advised."
6. If a shock is advised, press the AED shock button. As soon as the shock is discharged, immediately resume chest compressions and continue CPR for 2 min before doing a rhythm check again.
7. If the AED voice prompt does not advise a shock to be administered, resume CPR immediately.

3.4 Life Support Course Description

There are life support courses which have been developed by the American Heart Association (AHA), American Academy of Pediatrics (AAP), American College of Emergency Physicians (ACEP) and the Emergency Nurses Association (ENA). Table 3.1 summarizes thesec courses.

3.5 Teaching Office Emergency Preparedness and Mock Codes

Prior to instituting an office medical emergency preparedness and mock code program you must first survey the education needs and the resources available to your learners. Determine the common pediatric emergencies in their practice. These will usually include respiratory distress (due to asthma, bronchiolitis, pneumonia, croup), shock (due to dehydration, sepsis or anaphylaxis), seizures and choking. Find out the type of emergency supplies (crash cart, equipment and drugs, oxygen and suction) available and the number of health providers who are likely to be present. You should

Table 3.1 Life support courses

	PALS	PEARS	ENPC	BLS classroom	BLS online part 1
Overview	Classroom, video-based, instructor-led course Uses a series of simulated pediatric emergencies to reinforce the important concepts of a systematic approach to pediatric assessment, basic life support, PALS treatment algorithms, effective resuscitation and team dynamics	Classroom-based, instructor-led course. Teaches providers respiratory distress, shock and cardiac arrest, and provide appropriate lifesaving interventions within the initial minutes of response until the child is transferred to an advanced life support provider	Focuses on developmental, anatomical and developmental responses to specific pathologies of pediatric patients and provides critical integration of information essential to the emergency nurse	Focuses on the ability to recognize several life-threatening emergencies, provide CPR, use an AED, and relieve choking in a safe, timely and effective manner	Flexible training option Focuses on the ability to recognize several life-threatening emergencies, provide CPR, use an AED, and relieve choking in a safe, timely and effective manner Can choose this course for first time or renewal certification. Students first complete online lessons; then, meet with an AHA instructor for skills practice and testing
Learners	Healthcare providers who respond to emergencies in infants and children. Personnel in emergency response, emergency medicine, intensive care and critical care units such as physicians, nurses, paramedics and others who need a PALS course completion card for job or other requirements	Emergency medical technicians (EMTs), medical and surgical nurses, school nurses and any other healthcare provider who infrequently encounter critically ill infants and children	Registered nurses, with other members of the pediatric emergency care team invited to attend and test	Healthcare professionals who need to know how to perform CPR, as well as other lifesaving skills, in an in-hospital and out-of-hospital setting	Healthcare professionals who need to know how to perform CPR, as well as other lifesaving skills, in an in-hospital and out-of-hospital setting

(continued)

Table 3.1 (continued)

	PALS	PEARS	ENPC	BLS classroom	BLS online part 1
Content	• 1- and 2-rescuer child CPR and AED use • 1- and 2-rescuer infant CPR • Management of respiratory emergencies • Rhythm disturbances and electrical therapy • Vascular access • Resuscitation team concept • Cardiac, respiratory and shock case discussions and simulations • Systematic approach to pediatric assessment • Updates in 2010 PALS–AHA guidelines	• Pediatric assessment • Assessment and management of respiratory problems • Recognition and management of shock • Identification and management of cardiac arrest • Resuscitation team concept	ENPC provides education on triage, illness and injury, pain, airway, vascular access, critical care monitoring, resuscitation, trauma, burn and mass-casualty care, patient- and family-centered care, and medication safety Techniques for successful communication are included as they relate to each section, but are not taught separately	• Critical concepts of high-quality CPR • AHA chain of survival • 1- and 2-rescuer CPR and AED for adult, child, and infant • Differences between adult, child, and infant rescue techniques • Bag mask techniques for adult, child, and infant • Rescue breathing for adult, child, and infant • Relief of choking for adult, child, and infant • CPR with an advanced airway as an introduction to compression/ventilation rate and ratio for a patient who has an advanced airway in place •Updates in 2010 Basic Life support–AHA guideline	• Critical concepts of high-quality CPR • AHA chain of survival • 1- and 2-rescuer CPR and AED for adult, child, and infant • Differences between adult, child, and infant rescue techniques • Bag mask techniques for adult, child, and infant • Rescue breathing for adult, child, and infant • Relief of choking for adult, child, and infant • CPR with an advanced airway as an introduction to compression/ventilation rate and ratio for a patient who has an advanced airway in place. •Updates in 2010 Basic Life support–AHA guideline

(continued)

Table 3.1 (continued)

	PALS	PEARS	ENPC	BLS classroom	BLS online part 1
Format and theme	Full course: 14 h 10 min, Update course (with all optional stations): 8 h 20 min, Update (without optional stations): 6 h 20 min, Extra time for breaks	Full course: Option 1, following the BLS competency lesson = approximately 6 h; Option 2, with CPR testing during team dynamics practice = approximately 6.5 h. Update course: Option 1 = approximately 5 h; Option 2 = approximately 6 h		Initial provider course: 4.5 h including skills practice and skills testing. Renewal course: 4 h, including skills practice and skills testing	eLearning (online lessons blended with hands-on skills session) About 1–2 h to complete Part 1 Additional time required for skills practice and testing (Parts 2 and 3)
Features	• Course uses learning stations for practice of essential skills • Hands-on class format reinforces skills proficiency • Classroom-based works well for learners who prefer group interaction and instructor feedback while learning skills' • Co-branded with the American Academy of Pediatrics (AAP)	• Improves competency in pediatric basic life support • Learning stations and practice reinforce essential skills • Course video allows students actually see and hear critically ill children • Enhances skills in recognizing shock, respiratory failure, and cardiopulmonary emergencies	Online content, interactive lectures, psychomotor skills stations, case-based learning and small group discussions. The course includes a provider manual	• Video-based course ensures consistency • Instructor-led, hands-on class format reinforces skills proficiency • Student manual comes with new pocket reference card, designed to provide quick emergency information to the rescuer at any time • Updated science-based content	• Updated science-based content • Self-directed, Web based • Access to BLS for healthcare providers student manual • Downloadable algorithms • BLS for healthcare providers pocket reference card

(continued)

Table 3.1 (continued)

	PALS	PEARS	ENPC	BLS classroom	BLS online part 1
Certification	Students who successfully complete the PALS course, including the following components, will receive a PALS provider course completion card, valid for two years • Pass the 1- and 2-rescuer child BLS with AED and 1- and 2-rescuer infant BLS skills tests • Actively participate in practice and complete all learning stations • Complete the closed-book written examination with a minimum score of 84 % • Pass 2 PALS core case scenarios (1 cardiac and 1 respiratory or shock) as a team leader, providing appropriate medical treatment and demonstrating effective team dynamics	Students who successfully complete this course will receive an AHA PEARS provider course completion card, valid for two years	4 years	American Heart Association BLS for healthcare providers course completion card is valid for two years. In the classroom, students participate in simulated clinical scenarios and learning stations. Students work with an AHA BLS instructor to complete BLS skills practice and skills testing. Students also complete a written examination	Part 1 must be paired with a hands-on skills practice and testing session (Parts 2 and 3) with an AHA BLS instructor Students who successfully complete Part 1 receives a certificate that allows them entrance into a skills practice and testing session An AHA BLS for healthcare providers course completion card will be issued upon successful completion of all three parts

(continued)

Table 3.1 (continued)

	PALS	PEARS	ENPC	BLS classroom	BLS online part 1
Continuing education credit	Continuing Education Accreditation—Emergency Medical Services PALS course: 14.25 h PALS update: 6.25–8.25 h	Continuing Education Accreditation—Emergency Medical Services PEARS course: 6 h PEARS update: 5.5 h	16 h; No need for re-verification		
Source /URL	http://www.heart.org/HEARTORG/CPRAndECC/HealthcareTraining/Pediatrics/Pediatric-Advanced-Life-Support-PALS_UCM_303705_Article.jsp	http://www.heart.org/HEARTORG/CPRAndECC/HealthcareTraining/Pediatrics/Pediatric-Emergency-Assessment-Recognition-and-StabilizationPEARS_UCM_308135_Article.jsp	http://www.ena.org/coursesandeducation/enpc-tncc/enpc/Pages/Default.aspx	http://www.heart.org/HEARTORG/CPRAndECC/HealthcareProviders/BasicLifeSupportBLS/BLS-for-Healthcare-Providers—Classroom_UCM_303484_Article.jsp	http://www.heart.org/HEARTORG/CPRAndECC/HealthcareProviders/BasicLifeSupportBLS/BLS-for-Healthcare-Providers-Online-Part-1_UCM_303473_Article.jsp

base your curriculum on the American Academy of Pediatrics (AAP) recommendations for Office Emergency Preparedness and Pediatric Advanced Life Support.

If you wish to test baseline knowledge in pediatric emergency care, you may administer a pretest a few days before the mock code program (sample test included). The test may be sent electronically for ease of administration and analysis of results. A post-test can be administered shortly after the education program to improve knowledge retention among the participants.

It may be convenient to have the program last ninety minutes to two hours and to schedule it on a weekday during the lunch break to maximize participation and minimize disruptions in patient care. Alternatively, the program could be conducted after-hours.

Begin with a short didactic lecture of around 30 min. You could use a Power Point presentation on a laptop computer or project it on a larger screen. This will enable you to review key emergency care concepts and skills and set the stage for the mock codes that will follow. You may discuss the following: recognition, assessment, and stabilization of a severely ill child with an acute medical condition, organization, role and responsibilities of all clinic personnel during emergencies, storage of and access to emergency equipment and medications and role of emergency medical services (EMS). In addition, life support skills such as oxygen administration, suction, airway maneuvers (head tilt, chin lift, jaw thrust), bag and mask ventilation, automatic external defibrillator (AED) use, intra-osseous access and rectal administration of diazepam for seizures should be demonstrated and discussed. Advanced airway techniques will require more time, equipment and resources. Learners seeking to learn or practice these skills should be advised to attend Pediatric Life Support Courses such as PALS.

3.5.1 Response Team Roles and Responsibilities: Learning Through Videos

All members of the office emergency response team should be cognizant of their roles and responsibilities during an office medical emergency to positively impact resuscitation outcomes. Videos of mock code scenarios showing incorrect and preferred methods of an office medical emergency response are useful tools to learn these functions and to model effective resuscitation team dynamics.

3.5.2 Mock Codes

The next session consists of "mock codes." Mock codes attempt to create the best possible learning experience by trying to approximate a real emergency situation but may be unable to replicate it. Here, participants are asked to "treat" a mannequin based on commonly encountered emergency scenarios in pediatric practice (List of scenarios enclosed). The educational construct focuses on the ability of learners to correctly assess and recognize an office emergency, seek help from other providers, obtain and use appropriate resuscitation medications and equipment, perform important life support skills such as airway management and vascular access, reassess the patient's condition, include the family in the decision making, and initiate transfer of care to emergency medical services (EMS). The important points to consider are as follows:

1. Select an appropriate date and time to schedule a mock code. Initially, this can be a planned event. Later, this can become a surprise event once the office staff has had a chance to rectify their deficiencies from the initial visit.
2. The mock codes should be held in the clinic treatment room or examination room where the emergency equipment is located. If the "emergency" occurs elsewhere, the "patient" must be transported to this room. Office staff must locate and use their own equipment during the mock code in order to simulate a realistic environment. However, if there is a problem with restocking due to cost or other issues, you may lend your equipment.
3. Choose a few scenarios such as septic shock with hypotension and seizures with respiratory failure. Other scenarios may be selected. You will need to pre-determine the sequence of events in the mock codes and write down or print them before commencing. This will serve as a checklist on which to score each participant and the team as a whole in the interventions they perform (sample checklists are included). Ensure that all office personnel participate.
4. Bring a portable infant mannequin and basic equipment to the pediatric practice ex. *Laerdal infant mannequin (Laerdal Medical Corp, Wappinger Falls, NY)*.
5. Learners should ideally be assigned to 4-person teams (one physician, one nurse, one assistant, and one office clerk) and assume roles based on their skills. The physician will be the resuscitation team leader and manage the airway. The nurse will attempt and assist with vascular access, administer oxygen and medications and procure supplies. The assistant will document medications administered and assist in procedures or interventions. Finally, the front office clerk will summon EMS, copy the medical chart, and provide parent or family support.
6. If possible, videotape the mock codes after obtaining permission from the participants. The tapes will be helpful during the debriefing following the mock codes.
7. You will need an assistant to help with the mock codes. One of you will determine whether the participants are performing the required actions in the mock code and will use the checklist. The other will be needed for trouble shooting and to videotape the event.
8. Begin the mock code. Present a case scenario and have the participants resuscitate the mannequin. Observe if they assess and periodically reassess their "patient." They may ask questions to determine whether their interventions have been effective. If you notice that they arrive at a block and are uncertain how to proceed, you may provide an answer or hint. Let the mock code proceed allowing the participants to deliberate and work as a team. Do not be in a hurry to move to the next step in the mock code since you want to observe the time taken to obtain the equipment and medications and to assess the quality of their resuscitation skills.
9. The mock codes should be followed by a post-code debriefing session. Here, using the assessment tool (or video), explain where the participants encountered problems. This should pertain to actions such as identification of

abnormal vital signs, team dynamics, selection of appropriate equipment and medications, use of correct techniques for airway maneuvers and intra-osseous access, and adequacy of the end point of the procedure and mock code. Elicit their feedback and suggest solutions.

10. The mock code may be repeated to enable the learners correct their deficiencies. If time permits, a second mock code scenario may be presented.

11. The course may be more popular if you can apply for one hour of Category 1 Continuing Medical Education (CME) credit for the physician learners from the continuing education department of your hospital.

12. Mock codes should be scheduled periodically, probably every one to two years for best results (Fig. 3.3).

3.5.3 Sample Mock Code Scenarios

1. A 3-year-old boy with epilepsy develops a fever of one day duration. He is brought for a checkup. He begins to actively seize in the office waiting room.

2. A 14-year-old boy with a history of polyuria, polydipsia, and a 5 kg weight loss over the preceding 2 weeks presents to your office. He now develops repeated

Sample office emergency preparedness education program

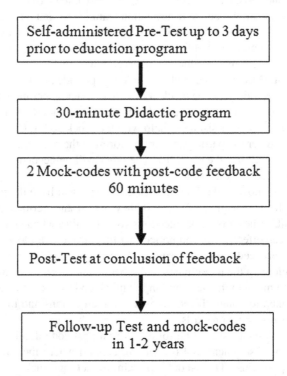

Fig. 3.3 Sample education program

episodes of vomiting and becomes lethargic and less responsive. His finger stick blood glucose is too high to calculate.

3. A 12-month-old infant has been having multiple episodes of diarrhea, almost one per hour, for the past 2 days. She is brought in lethargic with sunken eyes and tenting of skin. It is difficult to palpate her brachial pulses and she barely responds to stimulation.

4. An 8-month-old infant is brought to the office by his mother after she noticed a boggy swelling on the left parietal area. Her boyfriend stated that the child fell off the couch earlier that day onto a carpeted floor. The child is lethargic and there is bruising on the child's thighs.

5. A 24-month-old toddler picks outs a small toy from his mother's purse, puts it in his mouth, and then begins to choke. His cry becomes less audible and then stops. He appears cyanotic.

6. A 3-year-old child has been having a cough and fever for the past week. She is breathing very fast and grunting. A short while after you place her on oxygen, she becomes apneic. EMS has been summoned but has not arrived as yet.

7. A 13-year-old girl was stung by a bee about 30 min prior to arrival. She develops swollen lips, urticaria, wheezing and looks pale. She is having great difficulty breathing.

3.5.4 Mock Code Scripts (a) reactive airway disease/ pneumonia and (b) active seizures

This section contains scripts for two sample mock code scenarios: (1) Reactive airway disease with pneumonia and (2) Seizures. The script includes required interventions by each member of the office emergency response team (physician, nurse, medical assistant, and front desk personnel) and the "parent" or facilitator. Potential pitfalls during each step in management during the mock code are described. The teacher may use the mock code evaluation tool to assess the quality of emergency response and to provide feedback to each response team member (Table 3.2 a and b).

Table 3.2a Mock code script: Reactive airways/disease/pneumonia

Parent/Facilitator	Expected interventions			Front desk personnel	Pitfalls
	Physician	Nurse	Medical assistant		
Help me please!!!! I really need to see the doctor now. My baby is really pale and he is having a lot of trouble breathing. I can't wait any longer for my appointment				Yes I can help you (very calmly) Bring the baby in. (Receptionist calls for the nurse) Can I get an assessment to room one?	
Patient is a 12-month-old infant with history of fever to 103 × 2 days and cough, congestion, and wheezing		Bring patient to treatment			Failure to recognize a child with respiratory distress Inability to place the patient in the designated treatment area Inability to recruit the necessary personnel
	MD does quick evaluation of the baby Obtains a SAMPLE history	1. Quick nursing evaluation 2. Calls for MD		Stay with family to update about child's condition	Failure to evaluate patient and call for MD
A 12-month-old infant who lives with both parents and 3 school-aged siblings S: URI symptoms and wheezing X 3 days, fever to 103 but no vomiting or diarrhea A: No known drug allergies M: Xopenex 2 puffs every 4 h but it is not helping P: H/O RSV at 2 months requiring hospitalization L: last PO 8 h ago E: Continued fever to 103, increase work of breathing and wheezing despite ibuprofen and Xopenex treatments. Seems to be getting worse in the last 2 h Vaccines UTD	General: pale, crying, Temp: 105 C: HR 185 BP: unable to obtain Cap refill: 5 s, pale, cool to touch A: Patent, maintainable B: Respiratory effort: breathing spontaneously with coarse BS, diffuse wheezing, crackles RLL RR: 65 O2 sat 88 %	Begin documentation of vitals/interventions, etc Obtains vital signs; place on monitor (if available)	If nurse not available, begin documentation of vitals/interventions, etc		Failure to access CAB or vital signs

(continued)

Table 3.2a (continued)

Parent/Facilitator	Expected interventions			Front desk personnel	Pitfalls
	Physician	Nurse	Medical assistant		
	Calls for supplies Intervention: A: Suction airway, position head (head tilt/chin lift) B: Administer beta-agonist (Albuterol 0.083 % with 100 % oxygen) C: IV access, d-stick, laboratories Meds: Tylenol	Broselow® tape to determine weight/drug dosages RN #2: Begin documentation of vitals/interventions, etc		Calls EMS	Failure to call EMS Failure to use color-coded tape to obtain weight Failure to make airway interventions Failure to administer beta-agonist, incorrect flow rate or inability to connect mask to the oxygen source Failure to document interventions correctly
Reassessment: General: pale, increasing sleepiness C: HR 190, cool mottled extremities A: patent B: 58, severe retractions, O2 sat 89 %	*Reassess* Intervention: C: Unable to get IV access Attempt IO access NS bolus 20 cc/kg A: Airway maneuver B: none Administer ceftriaxone 50 mg/kg				*Failure to frequently reassess patient* Failure to reassess Failure to recognize worsening respiratory distress and pneumonia Failure to administer ceftriaxone Failure to progress to IO placement Failure to fluid resuscitate

(continued)

Table 3.2a (continued)

Parent/Facilitator	Expected interventions			Front desk personnel	Pitfalls
	Physician	Nurse	Medical assistant		
General: Unresponsive, pale/purple lips C: 205, mottled, cap refill 4 s A: patent B: RR 15, oxygen sat 88 %	Intervention C: NS bolus 20 cc/kg A: Suction B: Begin bag mask ventilation with 10-15L/min oxygen, one breath every 3 s, using the "E-C" technique to secure the mask to the face				Failure to recognize respiratory failure Failure to initiate BMV, Incorrect oxygen flow rate Incorrect mask size Incorrect technique to position the mask on the face
Reassessment: General: Responsive to pain C: 190, cap refill -4 s, mottled A: patent, maintainable B: RR assisted O2 sat 99 % with good chest rise	C: NS bolus 20 cc/kg A/B continue bag mask ventilation				Failure to administer additional fluid boluses
	Update EMS about patient Call the referral hospital and give report on the patient			Update mother about the status of the patient	Failure to keep mother update Failure to give report to the receiving hospital
	Lead debrief				Failure to debrief

(continued)

Table 3.2b (continued)

Parent/Facilitator	Expected interventions			Front desk personnel	Pitfalls
	Physician	Nurse	Medical assistant		
Mock code Script: Active Seizures					
Help me please!!!! I don't know what is happening but I think that my baby is having a seizure. She is shaking all over				Yes I can help you (very calmly). Bring the baby in. (Receptionist calls for the nurse) Can I get an assessment to room one?	
Patient is an 18-month-old infant with history of fever to 105. While in the waiting room, she began "shaking." Patient has rhythmic movements of both arms and legs		Brings patient to treatment			Failure to recognize a child with active seizure activity Inability to place the patient in the designated treatment area Inability to recruit the necessary personnel
		1. Quick nursing evaluation 2. Calls for MD		Stay with family to update about child's condition	Failure to evaluate patient and call for MD
	MD does quick evaluation of the baby Obtains a SAMPLE history				

(continued)

Table 3.2b (continued)

Parent/Facilitator	Expected interventions				Pitfalls
	Physician	Nurse	Medical assistant	Front desk personnel	
S: Shaking while in the waiting room, fever to 105	General: pale, unresponsive, arms and legs jerking, eyes deviated to the left	Begin documentation of vitals/interventions, etc	If nurse not available, begin documentation of vitals/interventions, etc		Failure to access CAB or vital signs
A: No known drug allergies					
M: Ibuprofen last 8 h ago	C: HR 185	Obtains vital signs; place on monitor (if available)			
P: No past medical history	BP: unable to obtain				
L: last PO in the waiting room	Cap refill: 3 s, pale, cool to touch				
E: He has had URI symptoms but no vomiting or diarrhea. Fever X 2 days to 105	A: copious oral secretions				
	B: Respiratory effort: breathing spontaneously with deep retraction				
	RR: 44				
	Air entry: coarse bilaterally				
	Calls for supplies	Broselow® tape to determine weight/drug dosages		Calls EMS	Failure to call EMS
	Intervention:				Failure to use color-coded tape to obtain weight
	A: Suction airway, position head (head tilt/chin lift)	RN #2: Begin documentation of vitals/interventions, etc			Failure to make airway interventions
	B: place patient on 100 % oxygen				Failure to administer oxygen, incorrect flow rate or inability to connect mask to the oxygen source
	C: IV access, d-stick, laboratories				Failure to document interventions correctly
	Meds: Tylenol				
	Diazepam PR OR				
	Valium/Ativan IV				

(continued)

Table 3.2b (continued)

Parent/Facilitator	Expected interventions			Front desk personnel	Pitfalls
	Physician	Nurse	Medical assistant		
Reassessment: General: pale, unresponsive, arms and legs jerking, eyes deviated to the left C: HR 190, cool mottled extremities A: copious secretions, upper airway obstruction B: 38, severe retractions, O2 sat 93 %	Intervention: C: Unable to get IV access A: Suction B: none				Failure to reassess Failure to recognize airway obstruction Failure to administer Diazepam after unsuccessful IV attempt Failure to progress to IO placement
Reassessment: No further seizure activity General: C: 156, mottled, cap refill 4 s A: copious secretions B: RR 5, oxygen sat 85 %	Intervention C: NS bolus 20 cc/kg A: Suction				Failure to recognize respiratory failure Failure to initiate BMV, Incorrect oxygen flow rate Incorrect mask size Incorrect technique to position the mask on the face
Reassessment: No further seizure activity General: C: 156, cap refill 3 s A: patent, maintainable B: RR assisted O2 sat 99 % with good chest rise	Administer ceftriaxone 50 mg/kg				
	Update EMS about patient Call the referral hospital and give report on the patient Lead debrief			Update mother about the status of the patient	

3.5.5 Mock Code Evaluation Form

Clinical Scenario _____

Date _____

	Yes	No	Comment
Obtains a sample history			
Clinical			
Circulation assessed initially			
Airway assessed			
Breathing assessed			
Initial CAB interventions made			
CPR initiated			
AED used			
Airway maneuvers			
Suctioning			
Oxygen administered			
BMV initiated			
IV/IO placement			
IVF administered			
Cardiac arrest board utilized			
Protocol followed			
Frequent re-assessment			
Secondary survey			
Medications administered			
Organization			
Patient moved to treatment room			
Personnel mobilized immediately			
Patient placed on monitor			
Emergency medical services called			
Broselow® tape used			
All supplies available			
Supplies located quickly			
Personnel used equipment appropriately			
Protocols available and used			
Resuscitation form available and utilized			
Communication			
Leader communicated effectively			
Events recorded accurately			
Roles were assigned			
Office staff called EMS			
Debrief session completed			

3.6 Sample Test for Training Evaluation

Check the **BEST** possible answer

1. A 10-month-old boy presents to your office with a 3-day history of diarrhea and vomiting. On examination, his vitals are as follows: temperature 99 F, blood pressure 69/50 mmHg, respiratory rate 40/min, and heart rate 168/min. The radial pulses are weak, and the child is drowsy. His capillary refill is 3 s. Which answer BEST describes the child's condition?
   (a) The child has uncompensated shock with inadequate tissue perfusion.
   (b) The child has uncompensated shock with adequate tissue perfusion
   (c) The child has compensated shock with inadequate tissue perfusion.
   (d) The child has compensated shock requiring no intervention.

2. A 4-year-old girl weighing 20 kg presents to your office with a petechial rash and has the following vital signs: heart rate 160/min, blood pressure 70/44 mmHg, respiratory rate 48/min, and temperature 104 F. She is lethargic and has a capillary refill of < 2 s. Her rapid bedside glucose level is 60 mg/dl. You decide to give her intravenous fluids. The MOST APPROPRIATE fluid to give the child is:
   (a) 200 cc of Normal Saline over one hour
   (b) 400 cc of D5 W 0.45 NS as a rapid bolus
   (c) 400 cc of Normal Saline over one hour
   (d) 400 cc of Normal Saline as a rapid bolus

3. A 2-year-old boy chokes on a small toy in your waiting room. He is coughing repeatedly; then his cough weakens and he becomes inaudible. You observe that he has no air entry in both lung fields. The CORRECT intervention is to:
   (a) Call 911 and give him blow by oxygen
   (b) Perform 5 back blows and 5 chest compressions
   (c) Wait for him to become unconscious and then administer bag and mask ventilation
   (d) Perform abdominal thrusts and reassess

4. A 5-year-old boy weighing 25 kg who was waiting in your office suddenly has a generalized seizure. He is brought to your treatment room while he is seizing. He has gurgling sounds and his lips are dusky. The correct INITIAL intervention is:
   (a) Start an intravenous line and administer 2.5 mg of diazepam
   (b) Call 911, administer oxygen and wait for the seizure to stop
   (c) Insert an intra-osseous (IO) needle and administer 2.5 mg diazepam IO
   (d) Place him in a recovery position, administer blow by oxygen, and use a portable suction to remove his secretions

5. A 15-year-old girl weighing 60 kg arrives at your office for treatment of a bee sting that she sustained just 30 min earlier. At the triage desk, she appears diaphoretic and pale. She is wheezing with oxygen saturations of 86 % on room air. Her heart rate is 126/min and blood pressure is 76 mmHg systolic. The correct INITIAL response is to:
   (a) Administer 2.5 mg nebulized albuterol solution in 3 cc saline
   (b) Give her an oral dose of 60 mg prednisone

(c) Administer 0.3 cc of 1:1000 epinephrine intramuscularly

(d) Administer 25 mg of diphenhydramine *(Benadryl^R)* intravenously

6. You decide to insert an intra-osseous (IO) needle into the tibia of a 6-month-old infant with septic shock. Which of the following is the BEST sign to indicate correct insertion of the IO line?

    (a) Ability to move the needle easily once it has passed into the bone marrow

    (b) There is a pulsatile flow of blood from the hub of the intra-osseous needle

    (c) An increased resistance is felt upon insertion of the IO needle into the bone marrow

    (d) Fluids can be administered freely without soft tissue swelling around the site of insertion

7. Which of the following devices can assure the highest concentration of delivered oxygen to a 3-year-old boy?

    (a) Non-rebreathing face mask with oxygen reservoir and oxygen flow of 10 liters per minute

    (b) Simple face mask with oxygen at 10 liters per minute

    (c) Venturi mask with 50 % oxygen

    (d) Nasal cannula with oxygen at 6 liters per minute

8. You are urgently summoned by your office security guard to provide first aid to a 7-year-old boy who was struck by a car in the parking lot. The guard activates Emergency Medical Services. You rapidly assess the child. He is unconscious and not moving. His lips are blue. Vitals are as follows: respiratory rate of 10/min and heart rate of 120/min. The correct INITIAL action is to:

    (a) Perform a head tilt and chin lift maneuver to open the airway

    (b) Administer chest compressions

    (c) Ask your nurse to immobilize the cervical spine of the patient and you perform a jaw thrust

    (d) Immobilize the patient's cervical spine and administer mouth-to-mouth respirations both by yourself

9. In a 5-year-old child who is apneic and pulseless, and you are the ONLY healthcare provider present, you must:

    (a) Administer chest compressions and ventilations in the ratio of 5:1

    (b) Administer chest compressions and ventilations in the ratio of 10:1

    (c) Administer chest compression and ventilations in the ratio of 15:2

    (d) Administer chest compressions and ventilations in the ratio of 30:2

10. A 14-month-old girl presents to your office with a temperature of 39 C, respiratory rate of 66/min, heart rate of 136/min and increased work of breathing. She suddenly becomes apneic. You administer oxygen by face mask. What is the NEXT intervention that you will do?

    (a) Leave the room to call Emergency Medical Services (911)

    (b) Perform a head tilt and chin lift and commence bag and mask ventilation

    (c) Attempt a jaw thrust maneuver

    (d) Intubate the trachea with an endotracheal tube

ANSWERS: 1-A; 2-D; 3-D; 4-D; 5-C; 6-D; 7-A; 8-C; 9-D; 10-B.

3.7 Office Emergency Preparedness Education Program: Practitioner Needs Assessment Survey

---

Office Emergency Preparedness Educational Program: Practitioner Needs Assessment Survey

Page 1 - Question 1 - Open Ended - One Line

What is the name of your practice site?

Page 1 - Question 2 - Choice - Multiple Answers (Bullets)

Which is your profession?

- ☐ Physician
- ☐ Registered Nurse
- ☐ Lieensed Vocational Nurse
- ☐ Medical Assistant
- ☐ Secretary/Receptionist
- ☐ Other, please specify

Page 1 - Question 3 - Yes or No

Do you maintain certification in basic life support (BLS)?

- ○ Yes
- ○ No

Page 1 - Question 4 - Yes or No

Do you maintain certification in PALS, APLS, or PEARS?

- ○ Yes
- ○ No

Page 1 - Question 5 - Choice - Multiple Answers (Bullets)

If you are a physician, how long ago did you complete residency training?

- ☐ <1 year
- ☐ 1-5 years
- ☐ 6-10 years
- ☐ >10 years

Page 1 - Question 6 - Choice - Multiple Answers (Bullets)

Which of the following resources do you use during a medical emergency?

- ☐ Broselow Tape
- ☐ PALS card
- ☐ American Heart Association Resources
- ☐ TCH Pediatric Office Emergency Preparedness Handbook
- ☐ TCPA Newborn and Pediatric Resuscitation Poster
- ☐ None of the above
- ☐ Other, please specify

Page 1 - Question 7 - Rating Scale - One Answer (Horizontal)

Rate your comfort level with your role in managing an office emergency

Very comfortable	2	Comfortable	4	Uncomfortable	Not applicable
○ 1	○ 2	○ 3	○ 4	○ 5	○ 6

Page 1 - Question 8 - Rating Scale - One Answer (Horizontal)

Rate your comfort level with managing a respiratory emergency in the office

Very comfortable	2	Comfortable	4	Uncomfortable	Not applicable
○ 1	○ 2	○ 3	○ 4	○ 5	○ 6

Page 1 - Question 9 - Rating Scale - One Answer (Horizontal)

Rate your comfort level with managing a seizure patient in the office.

Very comfortable	2	Comfortable	4	Uncomfortable	Not applicable
○ 1	○ 2	○ 3	○ 4	○ 5	○ 6

Page 1 - Question 10 - Rating Scale - One Answer (Horizontal)

Rate your comfort level with managing a choking victim in the office.

Very comfortable	2	Comfortable	4	Uncomfortable	Not applicable
○ 1	○ 2	○ 3	○ 4	○ 5	○ 6

Page 1 - Question 11 - Rating Scale - One Answer (Horizontal)

Rate your comfort level with managing a septic patient in the office

Very comfortable	2	Comfortable	4	Uncomfortable	Not applicable
○ 1	○ 2	○ 3	○ 4	○ 5	○ 6

Page 1 - Question 12 - Rating Scale - One Answer (Horizontal)

Rate your comfort level with managing an unresponsive patient in the office.

Very Comfortable	2	Comfortable	4	Uncomfortable	Not applicable
○ 1	○ 2	○ 3	○ 4	○ 5	○ 6

Page 1 - Question 13 - Rating Scale - One Answer (Horizontal)

Rate your comfort level with performing airway maneuvers.

Very comfortable	2	Comfortable	4	Uncomfortable	Not applicable
○ 1	○ 2	○ 3	○ 4	○ 5	○ 6

Page 1 - Question 14 - Rating Scale - One Answer (Horizontal)

Rate your comfort level with performing bag/mask ventilation.

Very comfortable	2	Comfortable	4	Uncomfortable	Not applicable
O 1	O 2	O 3	O 4	O 5	O 6

Page 1 - Question 15 - Rating Scale - One Answer (Horizontal)

Rate your comfort level with inserting an Intavenous line (IV).

Very Comfortable	2	Comfortable	4	Uncomfortable	Not applicable
O 1	O 2	O 3	O 4	O 5	O 6

Page 1 - Question 16 - Rating Scale - One Answer (Horizontal)

Rate your comfort level with inserting an Intra-Osseous (IO) line.

Very comfortable	2	Comfortable	4	Uncomfortable	Not applicable
O 1	O 2	O 3	O 4	O 5	O 6

Page 1 - Question 17 - Rating Scale - One Answer (Horizontal)

Rate your comfort level with your knowledge of where emergency equipment and medications are stored in the office

Very comfortable	2	Comfortable	4	Uncomfortable	Not applicable
O 1	O 2	O 3	O 4	O 5	O 6

Page 1 - Question 18 - Rating Scale - One Answer (Horizontal)

Rate you overall comfort level with managing pediatric office emergencies.

Very Comfortable	2	Comfortable	4	Uncomfortable	Not applicable
O 1	O 2	O 3	O 4	O 5	O 6

Page 1 - Question 19 - Yes or No

Do you think that a mock code performed by a member of the Texas Children's Hospital Emergency Department would be beneficial to your practice?

O Yes
O No

Page 1 - Question 20 - Open Ended - One Line

What is the best time of day to schedule a mock code?

Thank You Page

Standard

Screen Out Page

Standard

Over Quota Page

Standard

Survey Closed Page

Standard

Chapter 4
The Office Preparedness Quality Improvement Project

In 2001, the Institutes of Medicine published "Crossing the Quality Chasm" which identified 6 aims for improvement in health care. Borrowing concepts from manufacturing and industry, leaders in health care began adopting quality improvement strategies to improve the care of patients. We recognize a need to improve primary care pediatric office preparedness for medical emergencies. While emergencies are not a common occurrence in this setting, when they do occur, healthcare providers must be able to rapidly and effectively assess and stabilize patients until appropriate transfer of care to emergency medical personnel service. Several key components are vital for good patient care: availability of pediatric-specific resuscitation equipment, training of staff regarding pediatric-specific life support algorithms, presence of established protocols for emergencies, and mock codes for continued education.

To systematically address these needs and implement change, we used a model for improvement, (AHRQ, n.d) which asks three fundamental questions:

- What am I trying to accomplish?
- How will I know that a change is an improvement?
- What change(s) can I make that will result in an improvement?

The most commonly used framework for trial and learning is the Plan-Do-Study-Act (PDSA) Cycle (Langley et al. 2009; National Health Services Institute, n.d) (Fig. 4.1).

PLAN:

- Determine the objective
- State predictions
- Determine Who, What, When, Where?
- Collect data that helps to determine what the needs are.

DO:

- Carry out the plan
- Document problems and unexpected observations
- Begin data collection

R. Shenoi et al., *The Complete Resource on Pediatric Office Emergency Preparedness*, SpringerBriefs in Child Health, DOI: 10.1007/978-1-4614-6904-9_4, © The Author(s) 2013

Fig. 4.1 Plan-Do-Study-Act

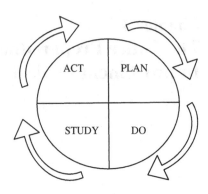

STUDY:

- Data analysis
- Compare data to predictions
- Summarize what was learned

ACT:

- What changes are to be made?
- What is the next cycle?

Here is an example of multiple PDSA cycles, in office emergency preparedness.

PDSA Cycle #1

PLAN:

- Problem: Offices are poorly prepared in handling office medical emergencies. There is suboptimal organization and availability of emergency equipment and medications

- Needs Assessment:
    - Emergency equipment
    - Emergency medications
    - Organization of both equipment and medications
    - Designated treatment area
- Specific Aim: Within 6 months of implementation

    - 90–100% of the offices will purchase the recommended equipment and medications
    - 90–100% of the offices will organize the equipment using either a cart or a tackle box
    - 90–100% of the offices will designate a treatment area for emergencies.

DO:

- Respond to resistance to change:

- Some practitioners may believe that medical emergencies present so infrequently to the office that there is no need to incur the additional cost of purchasing equipment and medications.
- Some offices may be in close proximity to a hospital;
- Some offices may be near a fire station; therefore, there is a short response time for emergency medical service.

STUDY:

- Measure the compliance in specific aims: What percentage of offices are able to purchase and organize medications and equipment and create a resuscitation area?
- Determine barriers to specific aims: What are the barriers to compliance?

ACT:

- Gather key stakeholders to review barriers to specific aims and create and implement solutions
- Perform mock code drills in 1–2 selected practices in order to gather data on deficiencies that can be improved upon.

PDSA Cycle #2

PLAN:

- Problem: Similar to cycle 1
- Needs Assessment: Similar to cycle 1
- Specific Aim: Improve knowledge, skills and comfort with management of various medical emergencies using mock code drills at 1–2 selected practice sites

  - Improve all the knowledge of the location of medications and equipment and designated resuscitation area to 100% of practitioners.
  - Improve practitioners' comfort in their role in office emergencies by 20–50%
  - Improve practitioners' comfort with bag/mask ventilation and effective chest compressions by 20–50%
  - Improve physician comfort in intraosseous (IO) placement by 20–50%

DO:

- Two mock code drills conducted either before office hours or during the lunch break
  - Two-person team (emergency medicine physician and nurse educator) present to the front desk of office with a mock patient having a medical emergency;
  - Instruct the staff to treat the mock patient as if it is a real patient.
- Conduct a de-brief session after each mock code drill.

STUDY:

- Assess mock code performance using a standardized evaluation form;
- Assess change in practitioner comfort in resuscitation after mock code;
- Identify specific gaps in performance and determine barriers to improvement;

ACT:

- Develop resource materials such as disease-specific management protocols;
- Expand mock code drills to additional offices;
- Create strategies for sustained improvement.

    - Checklists for equipment availability and maintenance;
    - Continuing education of current and new staff;
    - Create accountability by posting results of mock code drills and checklist compliance.

The framework listed above is meant to be a guide. It will need to be modified to suit each practice situation. The most important thing to remember is to identify what the needs are, determine what changes will constitute an improvement, and make small improvements in each PDSA cycle.

References

AHRQ Health Care Innovations Exchange. Qualtiy tool. Plan-Do-Study-Ace Act (PSDA) cycle. http://www.innovations.ahrq.gov/content.aspx?id=2398.

Langley, G. L., Nolan, K. M., Nolan, T. W., Norman, C. L., Provost, L. P. (2009). *The improvement guide: A practical approach to enhancing organizational performance* (2nd ed.). San Francisco: Jossey-Bass Publishers. http://www.apiweb.org/the_improvement_guide2htm.

National Health Services Institute for Innovation and Improvement. Plan, Do Study, Act (PDSA) http://www.institute.nhs.uk/quality_and_service_improvement_tools/quality_and_service_improvement_tools/plan_do_study_act.html.

Chapter 5
Family Education

Anticipatory guidance helps parents to prevent potential injuries and illnesses in their children and assists them in understanding how to navigate the emergency system if their child should require emergency care. The following instructions have been developed for parents whose children may encounter potential emergencies.

5.1 What to Do If Your Child is Having a Health Emergency?

5.1.1 What is a Health Emergency?

A health emergency consists of **an illness or injury that is immediately threatening to a child's life or limb**. These include a variety of conditions such as

- loss of consciousness or no response when you talk to your child
- seizures
- difficulty breathing
- severe burns (large, involve hands, feet, groin, chest, or face)
- ingestion of a poisonous substance
- severe injury from a motor vehicle crash or a fall from a high place
- choking
- vomiting after head injury

(Seidel and Knapp 2000; U.S. Department of Health and Human Services, Emergency Medical Services for Children, and National Highway Traffic Safety Administration 2012)

These are some of the conditions which require prompt medical attention since they can worsen.

Other medical conditions may not require emergency care. These include small cuts, fever in toddlers and older children, diarrhea or constipation, stomachaches, earaches, minor bruises, nosebleeds, rashes, or sprains. With appropriate instructions from your physician or nurse at the clinic or after-hours call center, you can manage these conditions appropriately at home.

Call 911 (or your local emergency number) for help if you are concerned that your child's life may be in danger or that your child is seriously ill or injured. If you are not sure that your child has an emergency condition, consult your doctor.

5.1.2 What Happens When You Call the Emergency Phone Number?

When you call the emergency phone number such as 911, a trained professional (emergency operator) will ask you a series of questions to assess your child's medical condition so that appropriate help can be sent to you. Do your best to stay calm and give the operator brief and accurate answers. This will help expedite the process. The operator may provide you with instructions on how to care for your child until help arrives. The emergency medical service (EMS) providers may also provide some medical care on the scene prior to transporting your child. While it can be stressful during these times, it is important to let the medical personnel take care of your child. They will do their best to keep you informed about present and future care that your child will receive (U.S. Department of Health and Human Services, Emergency Medical Services for Children, and National Highway Traffic Safety Administration 2012).

5.1.3 What Will Happen When You Get to the Emergency Department?

EMS providers have a good understanding of the treatment capabilities of the hospitals in your area. They will transport your child to the most appropriate facility based on the type and severity of your child's condition. Upon arrival at the hospital, your child will be reassessed by a nurse and assigned a triage level depending on the severity of his/her illness. Your child will need immediate care if his/her condition is critical. On other occasions, your child's condition may not be as serious and you may have to wait for a longer period of time before the doctor examines your child. Like your child, there are several other children at the emergency department who seek care. Waiting times can be long, so please be patient. The triage policy helps the doctors and nurses first identify critically ill children, so that they can receive timely care. In some instances, the condition of your child may improve during transport. The physician will check your child and discharge you from the emergency department. If your primary care provider sent you to the emergency department, the treating emergency physician will contact your physician to discuss your child's condition. If you have any concerns with the care that your child is receiving, please contact one of the nurses (U.S. Department

Table 5.1 Important numbers to know (keep posted near your phone or easily accessible area) (American Academy of Pediatrics (AAP) 2012)

	Name	Address	Daytime phone	Emergency/ after-hours phone
Child				
Pediatrician				
Dentist				
Emergency medical services (EMS)			911 (most areas)	911 (most areas)
Poison control center			800-222-1222	
Police department				
Preferred hospital or emergency center (discuss with your doctor)				

of Health and Human Services, Emergency Medical Services for Children, and National Highway Traffic Safety Administration 2012) (Table 5.1).

Resources: The following are sample resource sheets that you should strongly consider for your patients that summarize the information above.

- AAP handout: *When your child needs emergency medical services* http://www2.aap.org/family/frk/EMSFRK.pdf (*Accessed September 25, 2012*).
- NHTSA: *How to prevent and handle childhood emergencies* http://www.childrensnational.org/files/PDF/EMSC/PubRes/How_to_Prevent_Handle_Emerg_Complete__EP000576_1997.pdf *and* http://www.luhs.org/depts/emsc/preventbk.pdf (*Accessed September 25, 2012*).

5.2 What to Do Until Help Arrives

5.2.1 What is and is Not a Health Emergency?

A health emergency consists of **an illness or injury that is immediately threatening to a child's life**. There are a variety of situations that this would include such as

- loss of consciousness or no response when you talk to your child,
- seizures,
- difficulty breathing,
- severe burns (large, involve hands, feet, groin, chest or face),
- ingesting a poisonous substance,
- severe injury from a high fall or motor vehicle accident,
- choking, and
- vomiting after head injury.

(U.S. Department of Health and Human Services, Emergency Medical Services for Children, and National Highway Traffic Safety Administration 2012)

These are cases that will require prompt medical intervention involving specialized equipment, personnel and training.

Call 911 (or your local emergency number) for help if you are concerned that your child's life may be in danger or that your child is seriously ill or injured. Always remember that your pediatrician is available for consultation if you are not sure that your child has an emergency. While you wait for help to arrive, in certain situations, there are some steps you may take that could save your child's life.

CPR: One step you should strongly consider is taking a cardiopulmonary respiratory course. CPR is a simple skill set that you can easily learn that could save your child's life. CPR courses are available at many hospitals. The American Heart Association and your pediatrician can help you find a course in your area. Most courses last 6–8 h, teach CPR as well as first aid and ways to prevent emergencies.

The following are abbreviated excerpts from "How to prevent and handle childhood emergencies".

5.2.1.1 For a Poisoned Child

What you should do

- If the child becomes ill, call for emergency help immediately. If the child shows no signs or symptoms, call the Poison Control Center (PCC) as soon as possible for further instructions.
- Make sure to bring with you the container with the medication or product that your child ingested, inhaled or was exposed to when you call the PCC or when you go to the hospital.

What not to do

- Do not forget to bring with you the medication or substance that your child was exposed when you phone the PCC or when you visit the hospital.
- Do not give the child something to make him or her vomit.

5.2.1.2 For a Child Who is Choking

What you should do

- Call for emergency help immediately.
- If the child *can cough* or make any sound, do *nothing* until help arrives. If the child cannot make any sound and you have received training in choking management, you can attempt the appropriate technique depending on the age of your child.

What not to do

- *Do not* put your finger into the child's mouth if your child is still able to make any sound or cough or if you cannot see the object. You may make it get stuck or get further down.

5.2.1.3 For a Child Who is Bleeding Severely

What you should do

- Apply direct pressure with your hand, a gauze pad, or a clean cloth.

What not to do

- Do not remove any object that is in the wound.
- Do not probe or put any object into the wound.

5.2.1.4 For a Child Who is Badly Burned

What you should do

- Place a clean, cool cloth gently over the burn, then cover the child with a clean sheet and blanket for warmth.

What not to do

- Do not put ice, butter, or any cream or ointment on the burn.

5.2.1.5 For a Child Who is Having Trouble Breathing

What you should do

- Call for help right away. Allow the child to get into the position that the child finds comfortable.
- If your child is not breathing and you know CPR, start CPR.

What not to do

- If the child can talk or cough, do not take steps to relieve choking. Do not force the child to lie down.

References

Seidel, J. S., & Knapp, J. F. (2000). *Role of primary-care physician in EMS-C childhood emergencies in the office, hospital and community organizing systems of care* (pp. 27–39). Elk Grove Village, IL: American Academy of Pediatrics.

American Academy of Pediatrics (AAP) (2012). *When your child needs emergency medical services* http://www2.aap.org/family/frk/EMSFRK.pdf. Accessed 25 Sept 2012.

U.S. Department of Health and Human Services, Emergency Medical Services for Children, and National Highway Traffic Safety Administration (2012). *How to prevent and handle childhood emergencies*.http://www.childrensnational.org/files/PDF/EMSC/PubRes/How_to_Prevent_Handle_Emerg_Complete__EP000576_1997.pdf *and* http://www.luhs.org/depts/emsc/prevent bk.pdf. Accessed 25 Sept 2012.

Appendix

R. Shenoi et al., *The Complete Resource on Pediatric Office
Emergency Preparedness*, SpringerBriefs in Child Health,
DOI: 10.1007/978-1-4614-6904-9, © The Author(s) 2013

Important!
In order to be legally valid this form MUST
be printed on yellow paper prior to being
completed. EMS and medical personnel
are only required to honor the form if it is
printed on yellow paper.

This box will not show up when the form is
printed.

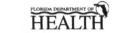

FLORIDA DEPARTMENT OF
HEALTH

State of Florida
DO NOT RESUSCITATE ORDER

(please use ink)

Patient's Full Legal Name: _____ Date: _____
                                   (Print or Type Name)

PATIENT'S STATEMENT

Based upon informed consent, I, the undersigned, hereby direct that CPR be withheld or withdrawn.
(If not signed by patient, check applicable box):

❑ Surrogate   ❑ Proxy (both as defined in Chapter 765, F.S.)
❑ Court appointed guardian   ❑ Durable power of attorney (pursuant to Chapter 709, F.S.)

_____   _____
(Applicable Signature)   (Print or Type Name)

PHYSICIAN'S STATEMENT

I, the undersigned, a physician licensed pursuant to Chapter 458 or 459, F.S., am the physician of the
patient named above. I hereby direct the withholding or withdrawing of cardiopulmonary resuscitation
(artificial ventilation, cardiac compression, endotracheal intubation and defibrillation) from the patient
in the event of the patient's cardiac or respiratory arrest.

_____   _____
(Signature of Physician)   (Date)   Telephone Number (Emergency)

_____   _____
(Print or Type Name)   (Physician's Medical License Number)

DH Form 1896, Revised December 2002

- -

PHYSICIAN'S STATEMENT

I, the undersigned, a physician licensed pursuant to Chapter 458
or 459, F.S., am the physician of the patient named above.
I hereby direct the withholding or withdrawing of cardiopulmonary
resuscitation (artificial ventilation, cardiac compression,
endotracheal intubation and defibrillation) from the patient in the
event of the patient's cardiac or respiratory arrest.

_____
(Signature of Physician)   (Date)   Telephone Number (Emergency)

_____
(Print or Type Name)   (Physician's Medical License Number)

DH Form 1896,Revised December 2002

FLORIDA DEPARTMENT OF
HEALTH
State of Florida
DO NOT RESUSCITATE ORDER

Patient's Full Legal Name (Print or Type)   (Date)

PATIENT'S STATEMENT
Based upon informed consent, I, the undersigned,hereby direct that CPR
be withheld or withdrawn. **(If not signed by patient, check applicable box):**
❑ Surrogate
❑ Proxy (both as defined in Chapter 765, F.S.)
❑ Court appointed guardian
❑ Durable power of attorney (pursuant to Chapter 709, F.S.)

_____
(Applicable Signature)   (Print or Type Name)

Date: Sept. 2004   Page 1 of 4

Do-Not-Resuscitate

Purpose: The purpose of this policy is to provide a guideline to prehospital providers, who under certain circumstances may accommodate patients who do not wish to receive and/or may not benefit from cardiopulmonary resuscitation. This policy is drafted in accordance with Public Act 368 of 1978, as amended, as well as Act 192 and 193 of the Public Acts of 1996. This policy is intended to facilitate kind, humane, and compassionate service for patients who have executed a valid "Do-not-resuscitate order" under the aforementioned Acts.

1. **Definitions**
    a. Attending Physician – means the physician who has primary responsibility for the treatment and care of a declarant.
    b. Declarant – means a person who has executed a do-not-resuscitate order, or on whose behalf a do-not-resuscitate order has been executed pursuant to applicable laws.
    c. Do-not-resuscitate order – means a document executive pursuant to Act 193, directing that in the event a patient suffers cessation of both spontaneous respiration and circulation in a setting outside of a hospital, nursing home, or mental health facility owned or operated by the Department of Community Health, no resuscitation will be initiated.
    d. Do-not-resuscitate Identification Bracelet or Identification Bracelet – means a wrist bracelet that meets the requirements of Act 193 and worn by a declarant while a do-not-resuscitate order is in effect.
    e. Order – means a do-not-resuscitate order.
    f. Patient Advocate – means an individual designated to make medical treatment decisions for a patient under Section 496 of the revised probate code, Act No. 642 of the Public Acts of 1978, being section 700.496 of the Michigan Compiled Laws.
    g. Vital Sign – means a pulse or evidence of respiration.

2. **Procedure**
    A do-not-resuscitate order is applicable to all prehospital life support agencies and personnel. A do-not-resuscitate order may be executed by an individual 18 years of age or older and of sound mind **OR** by an individual 18 years of age or older and of sound mind, and adherent of a church or religious denomination whose members depend upon spiritual means through prayer alone fro healing **OR** by a patient advocate of an individual 18 years of age or older.
    a. EMS providers **shall not attempt** resuscitation of any individual who meets **ALL** of the following criteria:
        i. 18 years of age or older
        ii. Patient has no vital signs. This means no pulse or evidence of respiration.
        iii. Patient is wearing a do-not-resuscitate identification bracelet which is clearly imprinted wit the words "Do-Not-Resuscitate Order", name and address of declarant, and the name and telephone number of declarant's attending physician, if any. **OR**

Michigan Department
of Community Health

M DCH

Jennifer M. Granholm, Governor
Janet Olszewski, Director

Michigan
System Protocols
DO-NOT-RESUSCITATE POLICY

The EMS provider is provided with a do-not-resuscitate order from the patient. Such an order form shall be in substantially the form outlined in Annex 1 or 2 and shall be dated and signed by all parties.

b. A patient wearing a "do-not-resuscitate order" identification bracelet, or who has executed a valid "do-not-resuscitate order" form, **but who has vital signs, shall not be denied** any treatments or care otherwise specified in protocols.

c. If a do-not-resuscitate order form is presented and is not substantially in the form as outlined in Annex 1 or 2, or is not complete and signed by all parties, **resuscitation will be initiated** while Medical Control is being contacted for direction.

d. In the event care has been initiated on a patient, and subsequently a valid do-not-resuscitate order form is identified, and the patient meets the criteria in Item 1 above, discontinue resuscitation.

e. A do-not-resuscitate order will not be followed if the declarant or patient advocate revokes the order. An order may be revoked at any time and in any manner by which the declarant or patient advocate is able to communicate this intent. **Resuscitation efforts will be initiated** and EMS personnel shall contact on-line Medical Control to advise them of the circumstances.

f. A patient care record will be completed for runs handled within this protocol. The patient care record will clearly specify the circumstances and patient condition found by the EMS providers, and describe the do-not-resuscitate documents involved.

Michigan Department of Community Health

M DCH

Jennifer M. Granholm, Governor
Janet Olszewski, Director

Michigan
System Protocols
DO-NOT-RESUSCITATE POLICY

Date: Sept. 2004   Page 3 of 4

"DO-NOT-RESUSCITATE ORDER"

I have discussed my health status with my physician _____. I request that in the event my heart and breathing should stop, no person shall attempt to resuscitate me.

This order is in effect until it is revoked by me.

Being of sound mind, I voluntarily execute this order, and I understand its full import.

_____   _____
(Declarant's signature)   (Date)

_____
(Type or print declarant's full name)

_____   _____
(Signature of person who signed for   (Date)
declarant, if applicable)

_____
(Type or print full name)

_____   _____
(Physician's signature)   (Date)

_____
(Type or print physician's full name)

ATTESTATION OF WITNESSES

The individual who has executed this order appears to be of sound mind, and under no duress, fraud, or undue influence. Upon executing this order, the individual has (has not) received an identification bracelet.

_____   _____
(Witness signature) (Date)   **(Witness signature)** (Date)

_____   _____
(Type or print witness's name)   (Type of print witness's name)

**This form was prepared pursuant to, and in compliance with,
The "Michigan do-not-resuscitate procedure act".**

                                                                ANNEX 1

Michigan Department
of Community Health

M DCH

Jennifer M. Granholm, Governor
Janet Olszewski, Director

Michigan
System Protocols
DO-NOT-RESUSCITATE POLICY

"DO-NOT-RESUSCITATE ORDER"
Adherent of Church or Religious Denomination

I request that in the event my heart and breathing should stop, no person shall attempt to resuscitate me.

This order is in effect until it is revoked by me.

Being of sound mind, I voluntarily execute this order, and I understand its full import.

_____   _____
(Declarant's signature)   (Date)

_____
(Type or print declarant's full name)

_____   _____
(Signature of person who signed for   (Date)
declarant, if applicable)

_____
(Type or print full name)

ATTESTATION OF WITNESSES

The individual who has executed this order appears to be of sound mind, and under no duress, fraud, or undue influence. Upon executing this order, the individual has (has not) received an identification bracelet.

_____   _____
(Witness signature) (Date)   **(Witness signature)** (Date)

_____   _____
(Type or print witness's name)   (Type of print witness's name)

This form was prepared pursuant to, and in compliance with,
The "Michigan do-not-resuscitate procedure act".

ANNEX 2

Michigan Department
of Community Health

Jennifer M. Granholm, Governor
Janet Olszewski, Director

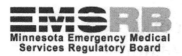

Minnesota Emergency Medical Services Regulatory Board

2829 University Ave. S.E., Suite 310
Minneapolis, MN 55414-3222
(651) 201-2800 (800) 747-2011 FAX (651) 201-2812 TTY (800) 627-3529
www.emsrb.state.mn.us

No Cardiopulmonary Resuscitation (CPR)

It is my/our wish that no Cardiopulmonary Resuscitation (CPR) be performed on:

_____

Print Name of Patient

_____   _____

Signature of Patient or Responsible Party   Relationship

_____   _____

Address of Patient or Responsible Party   Telephone Number

_____

Date

Do not perform CPR on the above-named patient/resident at the request of the family or other responsible party.

_____   _____

Print Name of Attending Physician   Date

_____

Signature of Attending Physician

"To provide leadership which optimizes the quality of emergency medical care for the people of Minnesota – in collaboration with our communities -- through policy development, regulation, system design, education, and medical direction"
An Equal Opportunity Employer

State of New York
Department of Health

Nonhospital Order Not to Resuscitate
(DNR Order)

Person's Name _____

Date of Birth __ / __ / __

Do not resuscitate the person named above.

Physician's Signature _____

Print Name _____

License Number _____

Date __ / __ / __

It is the responsibility of the physician to determine, at least every 90 days, whether this order continues to be appropriate, and to indicate this by a note in the person's medical chart. The issuance of a new form is NOT required, and under the law this order should be considered valid unless it is known that it has been revoked. This order remains valid and must be followed, even if it has not been reviewed within the 90-day period.

DOH-3474 (04/09)

Figure: 25 TAC §157.25 (h)(2)

OUT-OF-HOSPITAL DO-NOT-RESUSCITATE (OOH-DNR) ORDER
TEXAS DEPARTMENT OF STATE HEALTH SERVICES

| Print Form |

STOP DO NOT RESUSCITATE

This document becomes effective immediately on the date of execution for health care professionals acting in out-of-hospital settings. It remains in effect until the person is pronounced dead by authorized medical or legal authority or the document is revoked. Comfort care will be given as needed.

Person's full legal name _____ Date of birth _____ □ Male □ Female

A.   Declaration of the adult person: I am competent and at least 18 years of age. **I direct that none of the following resuscitation measures be initiated or continued for me:** cardiopulmonary resuscitation (CPR), transcutaneous cardiac pacing, defibrillation, advanced airway management, artificial ventilation.

Person's signature _____ Date _____ Printed name _____

B.   Declaration by legal guardian, agent or proxy on behalf of the adult person who is incompetent or otherwise incapable of communication:

I am the: □ legal guardian;   □ agent in a Medical Power of Attorney; OR   □ proxy in a directive to physicians of the above-noted person who is incompetent or otherwise mentally or physically incapable of communication.

Based upon the known desires of the person, or a determination of the best interest of the person, **I direct that none of the following resuscitation measures be initiated or continued for the person:** cardiopulmonary resuscitation (CPR), transcutaneous cardiac pacing, defibrillation, advanced airway management, artificial ventilation.

Signature _____ Date _____ Printed name _____

C. Declaration by a qualified relative of the adult person who is incompetent or otherwise incapable of communication: I am the above-noted person's:

□ spouse,   □ adult child,   □ parent, OR   □ nearest living relative, and I am qualified to make this treatment decision under Health and Safety Code §166.088.

To my knowledge the adult person is incompetent or otherwise mentally or physically incapable of communication and is without a legal guardian, agent or proxy. Based upon the known desires of the person or a determination of the best interests of the person, **I direct that none of the following resuscitation measures be initiated or continued for the person: cardiopulmonary resuscitation (CPR), transcutaneous cardiac pacing, defibrillation, advanced airway management, artificial ventilation.**

Signature _____ Date _____ Printed name _____

D. Declaration by physician based on directive to physicians by a person now incompetent or nonwritten communication to the physician by a competent person: I am the above-noted person's attending physician and have:

□ seen evidence of his/her previously issued directive to physicians by the adult, now incompetent; OR   □ observed his/her issuance before two witnesses of an OOH-DNR in a nonwritten manner.

I direct that none of the following resuscitation measures be initiated or continued for the person: cardiopulmonary resuscitation (CPR), transcutaneous cardiac pacing, defibrillation, advanced airway management, artificial ventilation.

Attending physician's signature _____ Date _____ Printed name _____ Lic# _____

E. Declaration on behalf of the minor person: I am the minor's: □ parent;   □ legal guardian; OR   □ managing conservator.

A physician has diagnosed the minor as suffering from a terminal or irreversible condition. **I direct that none of the following resuscitation measures be initiated or continued for the person:** cardiopulmonary resuscitation (CPR), transcutaneous cardiac pacing, defibrillation, advanced airway management, artificial ventilation.

Signature _____ Date _____

Printed name _____

TWO WITNESSES: (See qualifications on backside.) We have witnessed the above-noted competent adult person or authorized declarant making his/her signature above and, if applicable, the above-noted adult person making an OOH-DNR by nonwritten communication to the attending physician.

Witness 1 signature _____ Date _____ Printed name _____

Witness 2 signature _____ Date _____ Printed name _____

Notary in the State of Texas and County of _____. The above noted person personally appeared before me and signed the above noted declaration on this date: _____.

Signature & seal: _____ Notary's printed name: _____   *Notary Seal*

[Note: Notary cannot acknowledge the witnessing of the person making an OOH-DNR order in a nonwritten manner]

PHYSICIAN'S STATEMENT: I am the attending physician of the above-noted person and have noted the existence of this order in the person's medical records. **I direct health care professionals acting in out-of-hospital settings, including a hospital emergency department, not to initiate or continue for the person:** cardiopulmonary resuscitation (CPR), transcutaneous cardiac pacing, defibrillation, advanced airway management, artificial ventilation.

Physician's signature _____ Date _____

Printed name _____ License # _____

F. Directive by two physicians on behalf of the adult, who is incompetent or unable to communicate and without guardian, agent, proxy or relative: The person's specific wishes are unknown, but resuscitation measures are, in reasonable medical judgment, considered ineffective or are otherwise not in the best interests of the person. **I direct health care professionals acting in out-of-hospital settings, including a hospital emergency department, not to initiate or continue for the person:** cardiopulmonary resuscitation (CPR), transcutaneous cardiac pacing, defibrillation, advanced airway management, artificial ventilation.

Attending physician's signature _____ Date _____ Printed name _____ Lic# _____

Signature of second physician _____ Date _____ Printed name _____ Lic# _____

Physician's electronic or digital signature must meet criteria listed in Health and Safety Code §166.082(c).

All persons who have signed above must sign below, acknowledging that this document has been properly completed.

Person's signature _____ Guardian/Agent/Proxy/Relative signature _____

Attending physician's signature _____ Second physician's signature _____

Witness 1 signature _____ Witness 2 signature _____ Notary's signature _____

This document or a copy thereof must accompany the person during his/her medical transport.

INSTRUCTIONS FOR ISSUING AN OOH-DNR ORDER

PURPOSE: The Out-of-Hospital Do-Not-Resuscitate (OOH-DNR) Order on reverse side complies with Health and Safety Code (HSC), Chapter 166 for use by qualified persons or their authorized representatives to direct health care professionals to forgo resuscitation attempts and to permit the person to have a natural death with peace and dignity. This Order does NOT affect the provision of other emergency care, including comfort care.

APPLICABILITY: This OOH-DNR Order applies to health care professionals in out-of-hospital settings, including physicians' offices, hospital clinics and emergency departments.

IMPLEMENTATION: A competent adult person, at least 18 years of age, or the person's authorized representative or qualified relative may execute or issue an OOH-DNR Order. The person's attending physician will document existence of the Order in the person's permanent medical record. The OOH-DNR Order may be executed as follows:

Section A - If an adult person is competent and at least 18 years of age, he/she will sign and date the Order in Section A.

Section B - If an adult person is incompetent or otherwise mentally or physically incapable of communication and has either a legal guardian, agent in a medical power of attorney, or proxy in a directive to physicians, the guardian, agent, or proxy may execute the OOH-DNR Order by signing and dating it in Section B.

Section C - If the adult person is incompetent or otherwise mentally or physically incapable of communication and does not have a guardian, agent, or proxy, then a qualified relative may execute the OOH-DNR Order by signing and dating it in Section C.

Section D - If the person is incompetent and his/her attending physician has seen evidence of the person's previously issued proper directive to physicians or observed the person competently issue an OOH-DNR Order in a nonwritten manner, the physician may execute the Order on behalf of the person by signing and dating it in Section D.

Section E - If the person is a **minor** (less than 18 years of age), **who has been diagnosed by a physician as suffering from a terminal or irreversible condition,** then the minor's parents, legal guardian, or managing conservator may execute the OOH-DNR Order by signing and dating it in Section E.

Section F - If an adult person is incompetent or otherwise mentally or physically incapable of communication and does not have a guardian, agent, proxy, or available qualified relative to act on his/her behalf, then the attending physician may execute the OOH-DNR Order by signing and dating it in Section F with concurrence of a second physician (signing it in Section F) who is not involved in the treatment of the person or who is not a representative of the ethics or medical committee of the health care facility in which the person is a patient.

In addition, the OOH-DNR Order must be signed and dated by two competent adult witnesses, who have witnessed either the competent adult person making his/her signature in section A, or authorized declarant making his/her signature in either sections B, C, or E, and if applicable, have witnessed a competent adult person making an OOH-DNR Order by nonwritten communication to the attending physician, who must sign in Section D and also the physician's statement section. Optionally, a competent adult person or authorized declarant may sign the OOH-DNR Order in the presence of a notary public. However, a notary cannot acknowledge witnessing the issuance of an OOH-DNR in a nonwritten manner, which must be observed and only can be acknowledged by two qualified witnesses. Witness or notary signatures are not required when two physicians execute the OOH-DNR Order in section F. The original or a copy of a fully and properly completed OOH-DNR Order or the presence of an OOH-DNR device on a person is sufficient evidence of the existence of the original OOH-DNR Order and either one shall be honored by responding health care professionals.

REVOCATION: An OOH-DNR Order may be revoked at ANY time by the person, person's authorized representative, or physician who executed the order. Revocation can be by verbal communication to responding health care professionals, destruction of the OOH-DNR Order, or removal of all OOH-DNR identification devices from the person.

AUTOMATIC REVOCATION: An OOH-DNR Order is automatically revoked for a person known to be pregnant or in the case of unnatural or suspicious circumstances.

DEFINITIONS

Attending Physician: A physician, selected by or assigned to a person, with primary responsibility for the person's treatment and care and is licensed by the Texas Medical Board, or is properly credentialed and holds a commission in the uniformed services of the United States and is serving on active duty in this state. [HSC §166.002(12)].

Health Care Professional: Means physicians, nurses, physician assistants and emergency medical services personnel, and, unless the context requires otherwise, includes hospital emergency department personnel. [HSC §166.081(5)]

Qualified Relative: A person meeting requirements of HSC §166.088. It states that an adult relative may execute an OOH-DNR Order on behalf of an adult person who has not executed or issued an OOH-DNR Order and is incompetent or otherwise mentally or physically incapable of communication and is without a legal guardian, agent in a medical power of attorney, or proxy in a directive to physicians, and the relative is available from one of the categories in the following priority: 1) person's spouse; 2) person's reasonably available adult children; 3) the person's parents; or, 4) the person's nearest living relative. Such qualified relative may execute an OOH-DNR Order on such described person's behalf.

Qualified Witnesses: Both witnesses must be competent adults, who have witnessed the competent adult person making his/her signature in section A, or person's authorized representatives making his/her signature in either Sections B, C, or E on the OOH-DNR Order, or if applicable, have witnessed the competent adult person making an OOH-DNR by nonwritten communication to the attending physician, who signs in Section D. Optionally, a competent adult person, guardian, agent, proxy, or qualified relative may sign the OOH-DNR Order in the presence of a notary instead of two qualified witnesses. Witness or notary signatures are not required when two physicians execute the order by signing Section F. One of the witnesses must meet the qualifications in HSC §166.003(2), which requires that at least one of the witnesses not: (1) be designated by the person to make a treatment decision; (2) be related to the person by blood or marriage; (3) be entitled to any part of the person's estate after the person's death either under a will or by law; (4) have a claim at the time of the issuance of the OOH-DNR against any part of the person's estate after the person's death; or, (5) be the attending physician; (6) be an employee of the attending physician or (7) an employee of a health care facility in which the person is a patient if the employee is providing direct patient care to the patient or is an officer, director, partner, or business office employee of the health care facility or any parent organization of the health care facility.

Report problems with this form to the Texas Department of State Health Services (DSHS) or order OOH-DNR Order/forms or identification devices at (512) 834-6700.

Declarant's, Witness', Notary's, or Physician's electronic or digital signature must meet criteria outlined in HSC §166.011

Publications No. EF01-11421 - Revised July 1, 2009 by the Texas Department of State Health Services   **Page 2 of 2**

Important Emergency Telephone Numbers
(Fill in the blanks with your local emergency numbers)

EMS   911 or Local EMS Access Number _____

Non-EMS Ambulance Transport Services

_____

_____

Pediatric Transport Teams

_____

_____

Referral Hospitals

_____

_____

Poison Control Centers

_____

_____

Helicopter Service

_____

_____

Police (non 911) _____

Security _____

Other _____

_____

Index